T

C   l
guide for health
professionals on cleft lip
and/or palate

o9

D0525579

Cleft care:
A practical guide for health professionals on cleft lip and/or palate

Edited by
Vanessa Martin
and Patricia Bannister

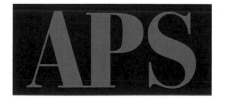

APS Publishing
The Old School, Tollard Royal, Salisbury, Wiltshire, SP5 5PW
www.apspublishing.co.uk   \00556244

British Library Cataloguing in Publication Data
A catalogue record for this book is available from the British Library

© APS Publishing 2004
ISBN 1 9038770 2 4

Printed in the United Kingdom by HSW Print, Tonypandy,
Rhondda

Contents

List of illustrations

List of illustrations

Contributors

Patricia Bannister, RN, SCM, HV, AdDipN, MSc, AdDip Counselling: Clinical Health Visitor Specialist and Lead Nurse, Manchester Cleft Lip and Palate Team; Nurse Advisor to the CSAG Committee; Chair of Cleft Lip and Palate Nurses Special Interest Group, 1999–2002; Convener and Practitioner/ Lecturer—Cleft Lip and Palate Nurses Course, Nottingham University. Nurse representative on the National Cleft Audit Group.

Lorraine Britton, MRCSLT, BA: Lead Specialist Speech and Language Therapist, Trent Regional Cleft Lip and Palate Team. Worked for 15 years as a paediatric speech and language therapist and for five years as a specialist speech and language therapist with children with cleft lip and palate in Nottingham.

Mr Mark Henley, MB ChB, FRCS (Ed.), FRCS (Plast.): Consultant Cleft Surgeon, Trent Regional Cleft Lip and Palate Team; Clinical Director of Plastic Surgery, Nottingham City Hospital. Trained in Nottingham, London and Miami. Civilian Consultant Advisor in Plastic Surgery to the Royal Navy and Regional Advisor in plastic surgery to the Royal College of Surgeons.

Vanessa Martin, RGN, RSCN, DPSN, MPhil., BA (Hons.), Diploma in Otological Nursing, ENB N.01 in Counselling: Nurse Consultant and Lead Nurse, Trent Regional Cleft Lip and Palate Team; Member of Department of Health Cleft Implementation and Monitoring Group; Convener and Practitioner/Lecturer - Cleft Lip and Palate Nurses Course, Nottingham University; RCN/Nursing Standard Child Health and Nurse of the Year Awards 2000.

Dr Donald H Rose, MB BS, MRCS, LRCP, FRCR, DMRD, Consultant Radiologist, Nottingham City Hospital NHS Trust since 1976. Formally research fellow in Ultrasound and Nuclear Medicine, Royal Marsden Hospital, London. Advisor to the Department of Health Cleft Implementation Group.

Gunvor Semb, DDS, PhD: Completed her orthodontic diploma in 1974 and joined the Oslo Cleft Lip and Palate Team. Since then, she *has worked exclusively with patients with clefts. In 1987, she became Director of the Cleft Dental Unit of the National Hospital, Oslo and was appointed Professor in 1995. She has participated in a series of international outcome studies on cleft lip and palate. She is presently Senior Lecturer/Honorary Consultant in Craniofacial Anomalies at the University Dental Hospital of Manchester and works in the Greater Manchester Cleft Team. She is the co-ordinator of an international multicentre randomised trial of primary cleft surgery.*

Bill Shaw *graduated in Glasgow in 1968 and has been Professor of Orthodontics and Dentofacial Development at the University of Manchester since 1983.*

He currently co-ordinates a multidisciplinary research programme on cranio facial anomalies for the European Commission, and the clinical section of a WHO programme on craniofacial anomalies. He is joint coordinating editor of the Cochrane Collaboration Oral Health Group.

Dr Mohnish Suri, *MD, FRCP. Consultant Clinical Geneticist with a special interest and expertise in dysmorphology, Nottingham City Hospital NHS Trust,*

Acknowledgements

Mandy J B Abbett, SRN, SCM, BFC: *Infant feeding specialist, with 19 years experience of teaching professionals and offering information and support to parents who choose to breast feed. At present working with Surestart, Chesterfield*

Sasha Andrews, Dip. IMI. *Medical Photographer, Department of Medical Photography, Nottingham City Hospital NHS Trust, Nottingham.*

Cathy Bown, DCR(R), DMU. *Consultant Practitioner (Ultrasound), Nottingham City Hospital NHS Trust. Responsible for a team of ten sonographers.*

Sara Deakin, RGN, DPSN, ENB 264 in Burns and Plastic Surgical Nursing. *Ward Manager, Adult Cleft Ward, Nottingham City Hospital NHS Trust.*

Mr Kevin Gibbin, MA, MB, BChir (cantab), FRCS. *Consultant Otolaryngologist, Queen's Medical Centre, Nottingham. He has a major interest in deafness in children and is the Lead Otologist for the Trent Regional Cleft Lip and Palate Team.*

Mr John E Rowson, BMedSci, BM, BS, BDS, FDSRCS, FRCS. *Consultant Maxillofacial and Cleft Surgeon, Trent Regional Cleft Lip and Palate Team.*

Foreword

Dr June Crown CBE

The lives of children with a cleft lip and palate and of their parents can be transformed by high quality care. The recent changes in the organisation of cleft care in this country aim to ensure that all patients benefit from the skills of the many professionals who can contribute to an excellent clinical outcome. This can only be achieved when these colleagues participate in teams where each member's contribution is fully understood and drawn upon throughout a programme of treatment that will last for several years.

However, professional and technical excellence alone are not enough. The child and the family, their needs, their anxieties and their idiosyncrasies, must always be at the centre of care. They must be informed about the nature of the problems and the options available for treatment. They must be able to participate in decision-making. The cleft team should aim to secure the trust of patients and parents and be able to demonstrate, through their audit and monitoring, that the care that is offered is of the highest standard.

This book emphasises the professional aspects of care, but never loses sight of the patient focus. It will help all those who contribute to cleft care to understand and appreciate the roles of their colleagues in the team. It describes the problems encountered and the interventions available at each stage of the patient's journey. It will also be of interest to the many parents who want to gain a fuller understanding of the condition and its management.

I welcome this addition to the literature on clefts and the help it will give to all those involved—professionals and patients—to achieve the shared aims of understanding and excellence in every aspect of care.

Dr June Crown, CBE: Vice-Chairman of the Clinical Standards Advisory Group Committee; Chairman of the Cleft Implementation Group

1
The service emerges

Vanessa Martin

Cleft lip and palate has traditionally been a service run by plastic surgeons and orthodontists, and was thought to be, primarily, to improve the cosmetic appearance for patients.

Over the last 20 years, the realisation of the importance of giving holistic care to the patient and family, has encouraged more professionals to be involved in cleft care. It is now expected that the service will be provided by a multidisciplinary professional team, which also includes nurses, paediatricians, speech and language therapists, ENT and maxillofacial surgeons, and psychologists.

Although individual units have, over the years, given a good service, in 1992, a European study indicated that treatment outcomes for children in the UK did not compare well with those in Europe. The study consisted of an inter-centre comparison of treatment outcomes of children with unilateral complete clefts of the lip and palate. It assessed the facial growth, dental arch relationship, and facial and nasolabial appearance of approximately 150 patients. It concluded that, in centres where there was standardisation, centralisation and the participation of high volume operators, there were good outcomes. In centres where there was non-standardisation and the participation of low volume operators, there were poor outcomes (Shaw *et al*, 1992).

Clinical Standards Advisory Group

As a result of this study, a clinical standards advisory group was asked, by health ministers, to advise on standards of care in the UK. This group was to review health care needs, clinical standards and treatment of children with a cleft lip and palate, and compare the effectiveness of high and low volume providers.

The group found that approximately 1000 babies were born in the UK with a cleft of the lip and/or palate (although the figures available were not reliable), that 57 units cared for these children, and 75 surgeons carried out primary cleft repairs. The majority of these 75 surgeons were performing only one or two primary operations on a unilateral cleft per year. They also found that 70 speech and language therapists were involved with children with clefts, 105 orthodontists and very few clinical nurse specialists.

Following these initial findings, 50 centres were asked to take part in a clinical standards advisory group outcome study. This was a retrospective study of the treatment outcomes of 457 children aged 5 and 12 years, with a unilateral complete cleft of the lip and palate.

A group of independent professionals assessed the following:

- **Dental arch relationship**, which describes the way the upper and lower jaw teeth bite together. *In 29% of children aged five years old and 34% aged 12 years old, this was excellent or good. In 37% aged five years old and 39% aged 12 years old, it was poor or very poor*

- **Alveolar bone grafting** was assessed based on a standard that every unilateral complete cleft of the lip and palate patient should have a bone graft to support the teeth by the age of 11 years. *They found one in six of children aged 12 years old had not had a bone graft. In the 42% who had, the bone grafts had failed or were seriously deficient*

- **The facial appearance** of 200 of the children aged five years old and 191 of those aged 12 years old was judged from photographs. *Fewer than a third of 5-year-old and a fifth of 12-year-old children had good or excellent lip appearance*

- **Speech** was assessed for intelligibility, consonance and nasal tone. *Nineteen percent of five-year-old and 4% of 12-year-old children were impossible to understand or only just intelligible to strangers. Only a fifth of five- year-old and fewer than half of 12-year-old children had normal intelligibility. Appreciable nasal tone was found in 17% of the five-year-old and 15% of the*

12-year-old children (which indicates a poorly corrected cleft lip and/or palate)

● **Hearing loss** and its nature was also assessed. *Twenty seven percent of children aged five years old and 18% aged 12 years old were found to have a conductive hearing loss.*

The overall results showed the UK standards to be well below the European standards.

The survey also looked at parents' satisfaction. The indication was that two thirds of parents felt that their child had received excellent care and only 6% were dissatisfied. The surgery of clefts is technically challenging and professional satisfaction is enhanced by the prolonged contact made between the cleft team, patients and the family. Parents could not be expected to know whether the best possible outcomes had been achieved, or the care that could have been provided.

Another survey by the Cleft Lip and Palate Association (CLAPA) also found high levels of satisfaction, but, at the same time, parents were concerned about lack of knowledge of the condition among non specialist staff and about poor co-ordination, communication and continuity of care. One in three parents were unhappy with the way news of the cleft was broken and more mothers wished to have the opportunity to breast feed.

It was not possible to fully compare outcomes of high and low volume providers because of the small number of high volume units and surgeons and because of poor overall results.

Conclusion

The Clinical Standards Advisory Group Committee recommended that future units should have two cleft surgeons receiving referrals of 80–100 new cleft cases of all types, per year. They felt that these numbers would provide the best opportunities for training, audit and research for all members of the multidisciplinary team. They recommended that surgeons, orthodontists, and speech and language therapists, who specialised in this work, should each undertake a minimum of 30 new cases annually (clinical nurse specialists will also follow this lead). They felt it was essential to provide a fully integrated multidisciplinary approach, centred on patients' needs from before birth through infancy, childhood, adolescence and to the end of facial growth. The cleft surgeon, orthodontist, and speech and language therapist would be joined by other professionals, including paediatricians, specialist paediatric nurses/health visitors, paediatric dentists, surgeons carrying out secondary surgery, geneticists, psychologists, ear nose and throat surgeons, and audiologists.

The committee recommended that surgery should be guided by protocols and that invasive treatment should not be attempted without a multidisciplinary review. Teams should take part in multi-centre audit and research, comparing programmes of care, and assessing parent and child satisfaction. These inter-centre audits require that centres should be large enough to provide meaningful data. For these audits to be performed, full records should be kept, including photographs, detailed anatomical drawings, and recordings of the child's voice. Cleft teams should also establish links with maternity units and obstetrics departments, in order to provide expert information as soon as possible after the diagnosis of a cleft. A clinical nurse specialist should be part of the cleft team that provides information and support—including feeding advice at the place of the birth and in the home.

The final recommendation was that a move towards between eight and fifteen multidisciplinary cleft centres nationally should be considered urgently, although additional centres might be needed for geographical reasons.

The Government response, when published, agreed there were too many centres offering cleft services, and that this resulted in poor standards of care and clinical outcomes for some patients. They proposed that, in England, the NHS Executive would set up a group to devise and oversee a strategy to implement the Clinical Standards Advisory Group recommendations (Clinical Standards Advisory Group, February 1998).

Cleft Implementation Group

In April 1998, a cleft implementation group of nominated professionals was set up to work in conjunction with the Department of Health. Their brief was to set out the arrangements for commissioning future cleft lip and palate services. Their work resulted in the publication of the Health Service Circular document entitled 'Cleft Lip and Palate Services, Commissioning Specialised Services'. This document (HSC 1998/238) (Department of Health, 1998) included the key responsibilities and skill mix of the main cleft lip and palate team to be based at regional centres, as well as the responsibilities of supporting services.

The main lead team, which was to see at least 80–100 new cases each year, was to be as follows:

- It should be led by a clinical director and should include:

  - Care coordinator/manager of the regional cleft service

  - Two lead surgeons who will each undertake primary surgery on an average of 40–50 new patients per year

  - Surgeon specialising in secondary surgery, such as bone grafting and orthognathic surgery

  - Lead orthodontist having a major commitment to cleft care

  - Lead speech and language therapist with a major commitment to cleft care

  - Lead paediatrician having a major involvement with the cleft team, ensuring good paediatric surveillance and ongoing paediatric care

  - ENT surgeon with paediatric experience

  - Audiological physician

  - Lead registered specialist paediatric nurse or health visitor with responsibility for providing feeding advice and support to parents, and the coordination of nursing activities

  - Appropriately trained psychologist.

It was recommended that, ideally, the main team should be based at the cleft or hub centre on one site. It was recognised that for reasons of geography and access some regions may find it necessary to have a main centre providing care on two sites. It was recommended that all primary and secondary surgery should be undertaken by a surgeon who is a member of the main team, at the hub centre within a paediatric environment. All care must be provided by paediatric trained specialist staff.

The extended team should include a geneticist, an ultrasound diagnostician, a paediatric dentist, a restorative dentist, and a maxillofacial and orthodontic technologist. There should also be a local regional parent support group.

Local or outreach arrangements should be made by the cleft team so that parents will only travel to the main centre for their surgery and specialist investigations. The main team may provide some outreach services on other sites, e.g. outpatient clinics. There should be good liaison with any extended team that may be in local centres. This extended team, like the main team, should be appropriately trained and accredited.

It was hoped that, by April 2000, the majority of regional centres would be allocated and ready to appoint staff, but the process has been slower than expected. By October 2003, the allocated hub centres at Birmingham, Nottingham and Cambridge; St Thomas', south of the Thames (temporarily at Guy's and East Grinstead); twin sites between Leeds and Newcastle, Great Ormond Street and Broomfield (north of the Thames) all had functioning teams. Twin sites between Oxford and Salisbury, and Bristol and Swansea are appointing staff to their teams. The remaining centre in the North West was still not allocated. It is hoped that all nine sites will be fully functional by April 2004.

2
Classification of clefts

Vanessa Martin

There are three main divisions in the classification of clefts. Clefts of the lip; premaxilla (primary palate clefts), and the hard and soft palate (secondary palate clefts). The junction between primary and secondary palate is the incisive foramen (*Figure 2.a*).

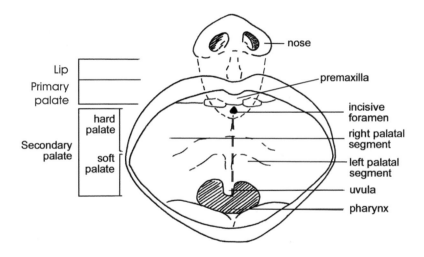

Figure 2.a: Classification of clefts of the lip, primary and secondary palate

Cleft lip (with and without cleft palate)

These can present as unilateral or bilateral, and incomplete or complete (extending into the nasal opening)(see *Figures 2.1.a to 2.6.c; Pages 8–15*). There is also a minor form of cleft lip known as a forme fruste, which gives the appearance of a scar (see *Figures 2.7.a to 2.7.c; Page 16*). The nostril on the cleft side is often distorted due to abnormal insertion of the obicularis oris muscle into the alar margin (see *Figure 2.b; Page 17*). A cleft lip can occur in isolation or in association with complete or incomplete clefts of the primary and/or secondary palate (see *Figures 2.2.b, 2.3.1.d, 2.3.2.b, 2.5.c, 2.8.a to d*).

Incomplete unilateral cleft lip

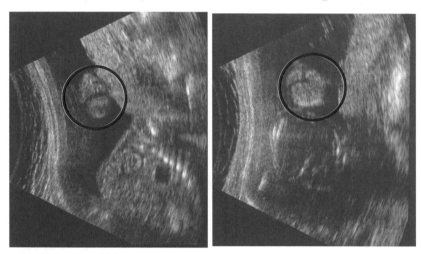

Figures 2.1.a & b: Two views of baby's facial scan

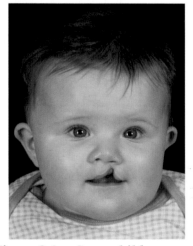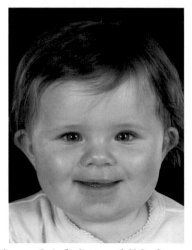

Figure 2.1.c: Same child as scan before surgery

Figure 2.1.d: Same child after surgery

Figure 2.2: Incomplete unilateral cleft of the lip and soft palate cleft

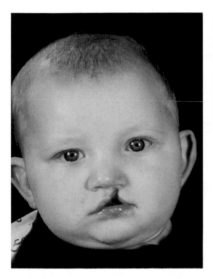

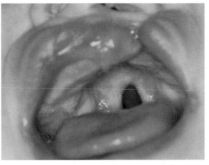

Figure 2.2.b: Same child's palate

Figure 2.2.a: Child's cleft lip

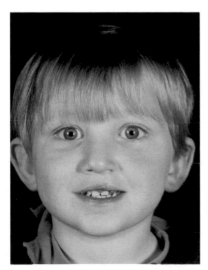

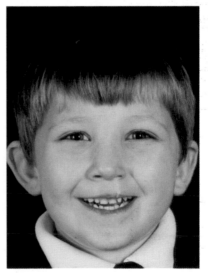

Figure 2.2.d: and at 7 years

Figure 2.2.c: Follow up views at
5 years

Firgure 2.3.1: Complete unilateral cleft lip and palate

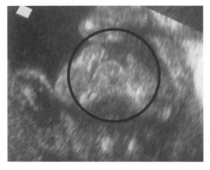

Figure 2.3.1.a & b: Two views of baby's scan pictures

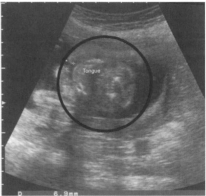

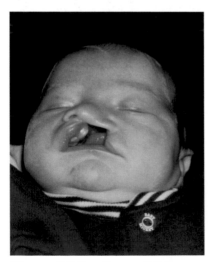

Figure 2.3.1.c: Same child as scan, before surgery

Figure 2.3.1: Complete unilateral cleft of lip and palate (continued)

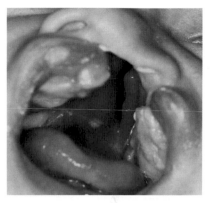

Figure 2.3.1.d: Same child as on Page 10, showing palate

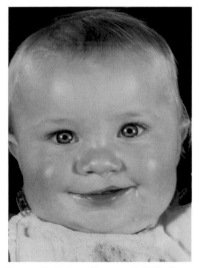

Figure 2.3.1.e: Same child after surgery, as on Page 10

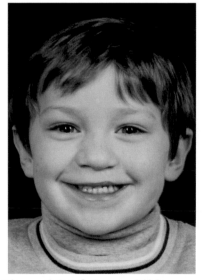

Figure 2.3.1.f: Same child, age 5 years

Figure 2.3.2: Complete unilateral cleft lip and palate

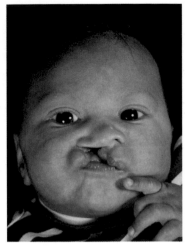

Figure 2.3.2.a: Child before surgery

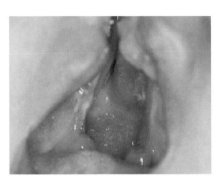

Figure 2.3.2.b: Same child showing cleft of palate

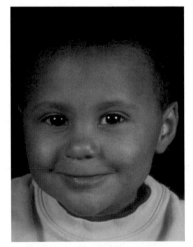

Figure 2.3.2.c: Follow up pictures at 5 years

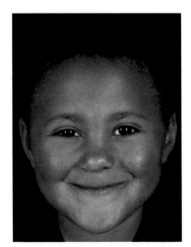

Figure 2.3.2.d: and at 7 years

Figure 2.4: Incomplete bilateral cleft lip

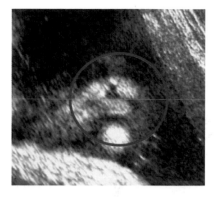

Figure 2.4.a: Scan picture

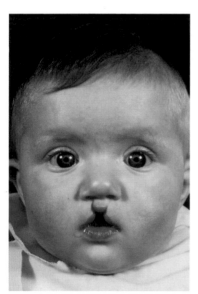

Figure 2.4.b: Same child as scan before surgery

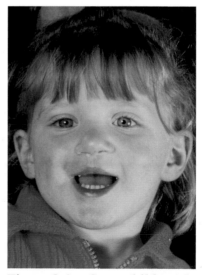

Figure 2.4.c: Same child aged 5 years

Figure 2.5: Bilateral cleft lip (incomplete on the left and complete on the right) with cleft palate

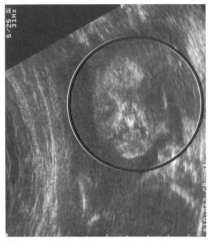

Figure 2.5.a: Scan picture

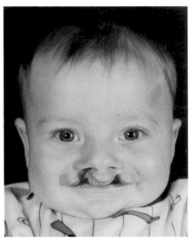

Figure 2.5.b: Child before surgery

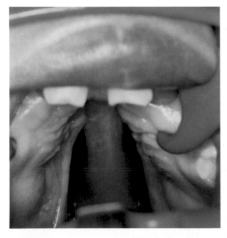

Figure 2.5.c: Cleft palate of same child

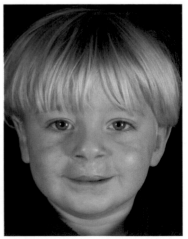

Figure 2.5.d: Same child after surgery, aged 2 years

Figure 2.6: Complete bilateral cleft lip and palate

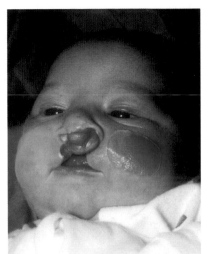

Figure 2.6.a: Cleft showing protrusion of the premaxilla (cleft of palate as child on Page 14)

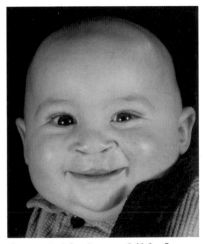

Figure 2.6.b: Same child after surgery

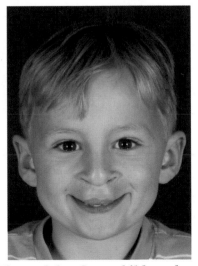

Figure 2.6.c: Same child aged 5 years

Figure 2.7: Left Forme Fruste

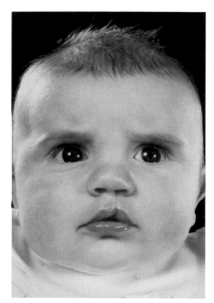

Figure 2.7.a: Child before surgery

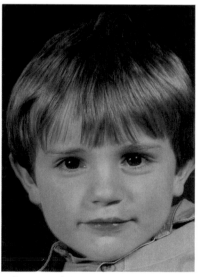

Figure 2.7.b: Same child after surgery aged 5 years

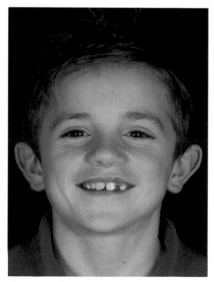

Figure 2.7.c: Aged 10 years

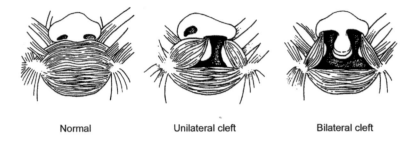

Normal   Unilateral cleft   Bilateral cleft

Figure 2.b: Abnormal insertion of obicularis oris muscles into the alar margin (From Management of Cleft Lip and Palate, Watson *et al*, eds. 2001; by permission of Whurr Publishers, London)

Cleft palate

Isolated clefts of the palate involve the hard and soft palates to varying degrees (see *Figures 2.8.a to 2.8.d; Page 18–19*). In all types of clefts of the palate, there is an abnormal orientation of the tensor and levator palatii muscles, which are orientated longitudinally and insert on to the posterior margin of the palatal bone, and along the margin of the bony cleft (Millard, 1980) (see *Figures 2.c* and *2.d; Page 20*).

Isolated clefts of the palate are often missed at birth, resulting in feeding problems and subsequent weight loss. Careful inspection of the palate using a torch and examination using a finger or spatula will enable the palate to be viewed as far back as the uvula.

A submucous cleft of the palate occurs when there is imperfect muscle union across the velum, but an intact mucosal surface (see *Figure 2.8.d; Page 19*). These clefts are frequently not diagnosed until the child presents with speech problems and may not be referred until the child is eight or nine years of age, when abnormal speech patterns are difficult to reverse. At birth, a bifid uvula can indicate that a sub-mucous cleft is present (although this is normally present in 2–4% of the population(Shprintzen *et al*, 1985)) (see *Figure 2.8.e; Page 19*). On palpation of the palate, a triangular notch at the junction of the hard and soft palate with a central channel down to the uvula may be felt. This central channel may be observed as a thin translucent area if viewed with a torch. Other symptoms, such as nasal regurgitation of milk, difficulty with the child taking his or her required volumes, or poor weight gain, may be other indicators of this condition.

Figure 2.8: Isolated clefts of the palate

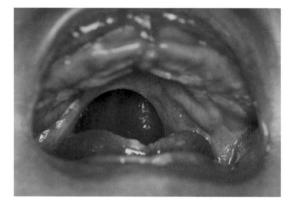

Figure 2.8.a: Horseshoe cleft

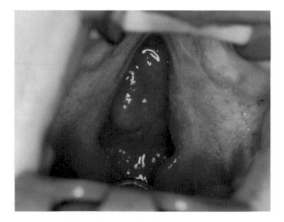

Figure 2.8.b: V shaped cleft

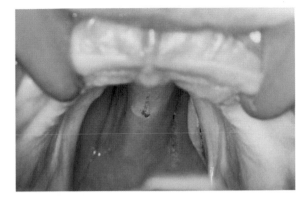

Figure 2.8.c: U shaped cleft

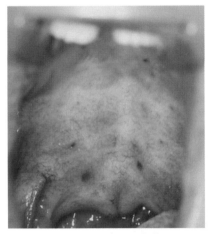

Figure 2.8.d: Submucous cleft

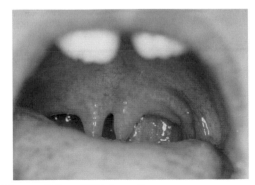

Figure 2.8.e: Bifid uvula

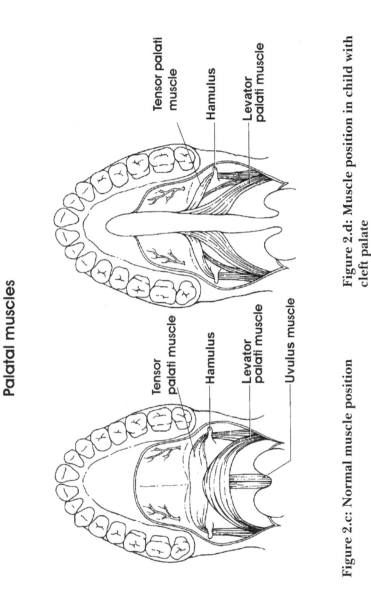

Palatal muscles

Tensor palati muscle

Hamulus

Levator palati muscle

Uvulus muscle

Tensor palati muscle

Hamulus

Levator palati muscle

Figure 2.c: Normal muscle position

Figure 2.d: Muscle position in child with cleft palate

3
Development of the face and palate and clinical implications

Vanessa Martin and Mohnish Suri

The development of the face begins in the embryo at the end of the fourth week, when the facial prominences, formed mainly by the first pair of pharyngeal arches, appear.

At four and a half weeks, the frontonasal, maxillary and mandibular prominences are the first to be distinguished, followed by the nasal prominences which form from the fronto nasal prominence (*Figures 3.a* and *3.b: Page 22*). By the end of the sixth week, the maxillary prominences increase in size and grow

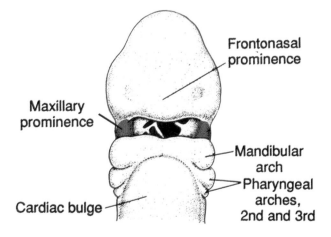

Figure 3.a: Frontonasal, maxillary and mandibular prominences

forwards compressing the medial nasal prominence towards the mid-line. The two fuse to form the upper lip (*Figures 3.b* and *3.c*; *Page 22*). Later, the maxillary and lateral nasal prominences

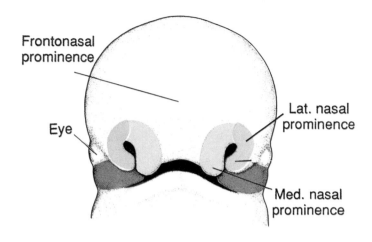

Figures 3.b: Nasal prominences

merge with each other and the maxillary prominence enlarges to form the cheeks and the maxilla (*Figures 3.d* and *3.e*; *Page 22/23*). At a deeper level, both the maxillary and medial nasal prominences fuse to form the intermaxillary segment. This segment forms the philtrum of the lip, and the median part of the maxillary bone with the four incisor teeth (*Figures 3.e* and *3.f*; *Page 23*). This triangular segment behind the lip is known as the

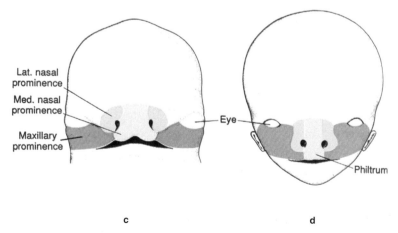

Figures 3.c and 3.d: Development of the upper lip and nose

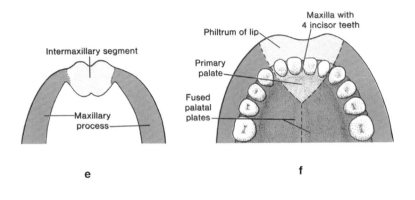

e   f

Figures 3.e and 3.f: Development of the primary palate and maxilla

primary palate. If there is failure in this fusion, an incomplete or complete cleft of the lip and the primary palate may occur.

Secondary palate

At the end of the sixth week of the development of the embryo, the secondary palate begins to form. The main part develops from two shelf-like out growths called palatine shelves which form from the maxillary prominences. These develop inwards and obliquely downwards on either side of the tongue (*Figures 3.g* and *3.h, Page 24*). The tongue moves downwards as the palatine shelves elevate into a more horizontal plane *(Figures 3.i* and *3.j; Page 24)* and by the end of the eighth week, have made contact, with fusion proceeding from front to back.

The process is completed by the eleventh week, although it occurs slightly earlier in males than females, (Burdi, 1969; Farrell and Holders, 1992). At the same time as the secondary palate is forming, the nasal septums grow downwards, fusing with it in the midline, to complete the separation of the two nasal cavities (*Figures 3.k* and *3.l; Page 25*) (Patten, 1976).

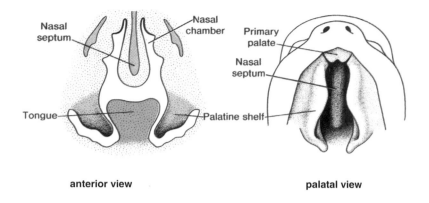

Figures 3.g and 3.h: Week 6 of the development of the secondary palate

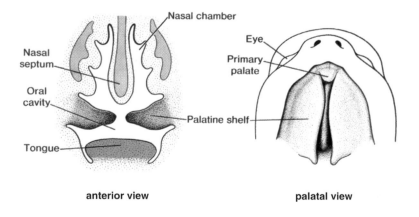

Figures 3.i and 3.j: Week 8 of the development of the secondary palate

The incisive foramen is considered the dividing landmark between the primary and secondary palates.

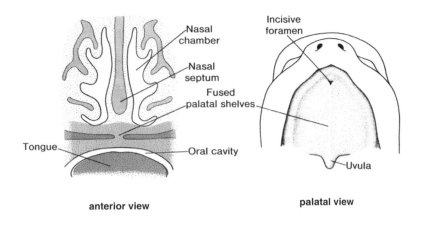

anterior view   palatal view

Figure 3.k and 3.l: Week 11 of the development of the secondary palate (Figures 3.a to 3.l: Development of the Face; modified after Patten 1976; by permission of McGraw Hill Book Company)

Epidemiology

Cleft lip and palate occurs in about 1 in 1000 white births (Derijcke *et al*, 1996; Harper, 2003). The prevalence of cleft lip and palate in Native Americans appears to be the highest of any group in the world. It is also high in Japanese and Chinese communities, but lower among blacks and Maoris (Croen *et al*, 1998).

Males with cleft lip and palate appear to outnumber females, whereas females appear to outnumber males diagnosed with an isolated cleft palate. Isolated cleft palates appear to be genetically distinct from cleft lip and palate with a frequency of 1 in 2500 (Roberts *et al*, 1996), as siblings of patients with cleft lip and palate have an increased frequency of the same anomaly, but not of isolated cleft palate and visa versa.

Submucous palatal cleft refers to the condition in which there is imperfect muscle union across the velum, but an intact mucosal surface, and the incidence is approximately 1 in 1200 to 1 in 2000 births (Bagatin, 1985). In this condition, velo-pharyngeal closure is incompetent resulting in hypernasal speech. Kono *et al* (1981) estimated that about 13% of patients with clefts of the primary palate also have a submucous cleft of the secondary palate.

Genetic factors in cleft lip and palate

When considering the genetic contribution to cleft lip and palate, it is customary to distinguish between syndromal and non-syndromal forms. The term 'syndromal' indicates that a child's cleft is part of a more complex condition in which other malformations may be present. The data reporting the frequency of other anomalies associated with cleft lip and/or palate is inconsistent. Syndromal causes are reported to account for approximately 44% of all cases of cleft lip and palate (Rollnick and Pruzansky, 1981) or 60% (Shprintzen *et al*, 1985). These authors do not attempt to separate cleft lip and palate from isolated cleft palate where anomalies are more frequent. Syndromes can be caused by chromosome abnormalities, by defects in a single gene, or by non-genetic factors, such as (rarely) exposure to teratogenic drugs in pregnancy. The diagnosis of a syndrome will involve referral to a specialist clinical genetic centre, where a full assessment and appropriate investigations can be undertaken.

It is important to note that some syndromes can be very subtle in their presentation. For example, in Van der Woude syndrome, which can run in families through many generations, cleft lip and palate is associated with small paramedian pits in the lower lip. Velocardiofacial syndrome can also present with the isolated symptoms of velopharyngeal incompetence (VPI), which causes difficulties with feeding and with speech.

The remaining cases of cleft lip and palate are referred to as non-syndromal or uncomplicated. This means that the cleft is an isolated finding. The precise cause of non-syndromal cleft lip and palate is not fully understood, but there is good evidence that both genetic and environmental factors are involved. For this reason, cleft lip and palate is often said to be multifactorial in origin, and it is generally believed that several perfectly normal genes interact in an unusual way to convey a susceptibility, which is then triggered by hypothetical and, as yet, unknown environmental factors. One theory is that various genetic and/or environmental factors may inhibit the flow, or decrease the number, of neural crest cells, or effect their mass so that contact between the nasal prominences may be impossible or inadequate (Johnston and Sulik, 1979). Clefts of the secondary palate may result from either hypoplasia of the shelves or delay in timing of shelf elevation (Gorlin *et al*, 2001).

Table 3.1: Risks for cleft lip/palate in family relatives

Affective relative(s)	Cleft lip and cleft palate	Cleft palate
1 sibling	4%	2%
2 siblings	10%	8%
1 parent	4%	3%
Both parents	35%	25%
1 parent and one sibling	10%	10%
1 aunt, uncle, nephew or niece	0.5% (1/200)	less than 0.5% (less than 1/200)
1 first cousin	0.3% (1/3,000)	less than 0.5% (less than 1/200)
General population incidence	0.1% (1/1,000)	0.05% (1/2,000)

(Modified from Harper P S (2003). Practical Genetic Counselling, 5th edn. Butterworth Heinemann, Oxford)

Whatever the cause, the role of genetics is borne out by the study of the incidence of cleft lip and palate in close relatives of affected children. These studies consistently demonstrate that a close relative shows a much higher risk frequency than is seen in the general population.

Examples of risk figures, which are often used for genetic counselling, are shown in *Table 3.1*. When using this table, it is important to note that isolated clefts of the palate appear to be a separate entity from cleft lip with or without a cleft palate. Also, if a child is more severely affected then the risks to close relatives are slightly greater.

At the present time there are no molecular genetic tests available for identifying susceptibility to the development of cleft lip and palate, and it is unlikely that such tests will be available within the foreseeable future. Nor are there any proven methods for preventing the development of cleft lip and palate in susceptible patients. Evidence of the use of multivitamins and high dose folic acid in early pregnancy is controversial. Some data supports this contention in some cleft types (Itikala *et al*, 2001; Tolarova and Harris, 1995). Folic acid supplements taken by the mother before and during early pregnancy may, therefore, reduce the risks. However, more studies are needed to address this issue.

Syndromes associated with clefting

There are over 400 syndromes associated with clefting. Some of them are extremely rare. New syndromes are constantly being reported, so it is difficult to be aware of them all.

When considering syndromes and clefting, more malformations are associated with isolated clefts of the palate than with clefts of the lip and palate, and more in bilateral clefts of the lip and palate than with unilateral clefts of lip the and/or palate.

Congenital heart defects are found in 3–7% of clefts, (Fallot's tetralogy being especially frequent), 15–20% have vertebral abnormalities, and there is an increase in urinary tract anomalies (Gorlin *et al*, 2001).

The most common anomaly associated with an isolated cleft palate is Pierre Robin sequence. This is characterised by a U or V-shaped cleft palate, micrognathia and a posteriorly placed tongue, resulting in airway problems.

Table 2.2: Some common syndromes

Syndromes	Some characteristics
Apert	Craniosynostosis, prominent eyes, beak nose, fusion of digits and toes (mitten hands and feet).
Beckwith-Wiedermann	Macroglossia which may affect respiratory tract and lead to feeding difficulties, macrosomia, hemihyperplasia, hypoglycaemia, omphalocele, large kidneys and renal medullary dysplasia.
CHARGE association	**C**oloboma of iris/retina **H**eart defects **A**tresia of choanae **R**etardation of growth and development **G**enital abnormalities **E**ar abnormalities and deafness
EEC (ectrodactyly-ectodermal dysplasia—clefting)	Ectrodactyly (split hand/foot) can be accompanied by syndactyly (webbed digits) or oligodactyly (missing digits). Ectodermal part involves hair, teeth and nails
Goldenhar	Asymmetry of face, small ear with preauricular tags, ocular dermoid, cervical vertebral abnormalities
Larsen	Multiple joint dislocation, hypertelorism, flat facies with depressed nasal bridge
Oral–facial-digital	Midline cleft or notch of lip, with cleft of alveolus and palate, multiple oral frenulae, synpolydactyly of fingers and toes. May be short webbed fingers and toes, polycystic kidneys, learning difficulties
Oto-palatal-digital	Conductive deafness due to abnormalities of ossicles. Possible flattened ends of thumbs and big toes, and webbing of digits.
Stickler	Features of Pierre-Robin sequence at birth. Mid face hypoplasia associated with prominent eyes and small nose. Hearing loss. Myopia. Vitreous abnormalities leading to retinal detachment. Skeletal problems

Syndromes	Some characteristics
Treacher Collins	Disorder of craniofacial development including hypoplasia of facial bones and mandible, malformation of external ears and ossicles, coloboma of inferior eylids
Trisomy 13	Varying degree of holoprosencephaly, premaxillary agenesis, eye defects, polydactyly, skin defects of posterior scalp
Trisomy 18	More than 130 different abnormalities noted, including microcephaly, clenched hand, short sternum, cardiac anomalies. Poor prognosis—if survive more than one year, severe mental deficiency
Van der Woude	Dominantly inherited disorder characterised by pits/sinuses of lower lip
Velocardiofacial (VCFS) (22q11 deletion)	Commonly associated with isolated cleft palate or submucous cleft palate. Includes cardiac anomalies, learning difficulties, immunological defects (particularly of T cell production). Overlap with Di George (also 22q11 deletion)

(Gorlin *et al*, 2001; Jones, 1997; Lees, 2001)

4
Prenatal diagnosis of cleft lip

Vanessa Martin and Donald H Rose

The prenatal diagnosis of a cleft lip is becoming more frequent as detection improves with experience and better technology, but expectations of ultrasound should not be unrealistic.

Although examination of the foetal face is a component part of the current guidelines for the second trimester ultrasound examination (UK Association of Sonographers, 2001; Royal College of Obstetricians and Gynaecologists, 2000), many units do not include this in their routine scanning protocol. Restrictions of funding and staffing may limit units to examining for life threatening conditions or those pertaining to long term disabilities and treatments. These are essential reasons for screening.

Units that routinely examine the face still encounter many obstacles, which restrict the sonographer's view; for example:

● Maternal obesity

● Oligohydramnios

● Adverse foetal positions, i.e. face against mother's spinal column or placenta, head too low

● Hands, arms, feet or cord in front of the face

● Multiple pregnancy

● Early or very late gestation

● Skill and time limitations of the sonographer.

In these situations, it may not be practical to bring patients back for re-scanning unless there is a family history of clefting.

A sonographer, experienced in the prenatal detection of facial clefts, should be able to identify if the cleft is:

1)   lateral, or in the midline

2)   unilateral (*Scans 4.1.a; 4.1.b; 4.2.a; 4.2.b*) or bilateral (*Scans 4.3.a; 4.3.b; 4.4.a*)

3)   complete (*Scans 4.2.a; 4.2.b; 4.4.a*) or incomplete (*Scans 4.1.a;* 4.3.a; 4.5.c) (extending into the nostril or not)

4)   involving the alveolus (*Scans 4.2.a; 4.3.b; 4.5.a*) or not (*Scan 4.3.a*)

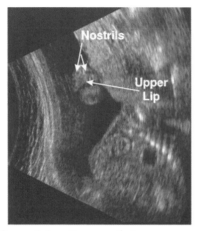

Scan 4.1.a: Incomplete unilateral cleft lip

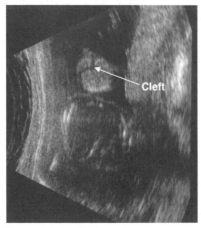

Scan 4.1.b: Incomplete unilateral cleft lip

It may be possible to show extension of a cleft into the palate (*Scans 4.2.b; 4.5.a*), but the clefts of the palate are very difficult to demonstrate by ultrasound, particularly in the absence of cleft lip. Midline (median) clefts are rare and are often associated with other anomalies, especially chromosomal disease.

The upper lip is best demonstrated in the modified (tilted) coronal plane, (*Scans 4.2.a; 4.3.a & b; 4.4.a*) and the alveolus in the transverse (axial) plane (*Scans 4.2.b; 4.5.a*). The sagittal plane is useful in the demonstration of the normal hard palate (*Scan 4.5.d*), of micrognathia, and of the abnormal pre-maxilla associated with bilateral alveolar clefting (*Scan 4.5.b*). Clefts of the hard palate may sometimes be seen in the transverse plane (*Scans 4.2.b; 4.5.a*). Colour flow doppler ultrasound in the sagittal plane shows fluid movement in the nose and the mouth. Lack of flow between the two helps to confirm that the palate is intact (*Scan 4.5.e*).

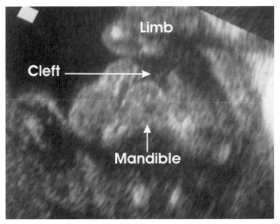

Scan 4.2.a Complete unilateral lip and palate: modified (tilted) coronal plane

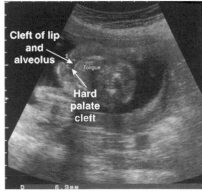

Scan 4.2.b: Complete unilateral lip and palate: transverse (axial) plane

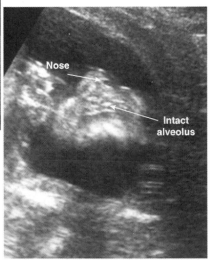

Scan 4.3.a Incomplete bilateral cleft lip: modified (tilted) coronal plane

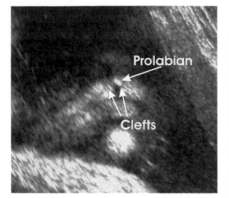

Scan 4.3.b: Incomplete bilateral cleft lip: modified coronal plane

The most important consideration when a cleft has been identified pre-natally is the feelings of the parents. Often, they will have no perception of what a cleft is (Martin *et al*, unpublished) and will imagine their baby to be grossly disfigured if they are not given accurate inform- ation with an appropriate information leaflet. It is im- portant that the sonograph- er confirms the findings with another experienced colleague before talking to the parents.

The Health Service Circular HSC 238/1998 insists that 'confirmation and classification of the diagnosis should be made

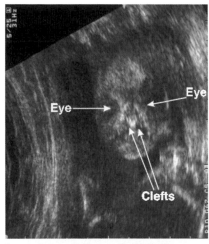

Scan 4.4.a: Bilateral cleft lip (incomplete on left and complete on right): modified coronal plane

by an ultrasound diagnosti-cian, who is either a member of the cleft team or who is recognised as having a special interest in prenatal cleft diag-nosis.' The Clinical Standards Advisory Group recom-mended high volume opera-tors to try to improve quality outcomes (CSAG, 1998). It is important to realise that a false positive diagnosis could result in the abortion of an unaffected child.

It may be appropriate to refer the mother to the local foetal medicine depart-ment for further investiga-tions, if other anomalies are demonstrated.

As soon as the diagnosis is given to the parents, a referral should be made to the regional cleft lip and palate team. If the parents have been told, and wish to know more, it is essential that telephone contact be made with the cleft team before they leave the scanning department, so that arrangements can be made to meet a member of the cleft nursing team and, if they wish it, a family with a similarly affected child (CLAPA, 2001; Martin *et al* (unpublished). Parents are very shocked when they learn that their

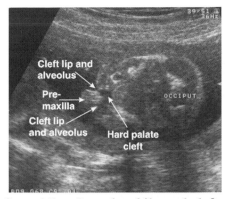

Scan 4.5.a: Complete bilateral cleft lip and palate: transverse (axial) plane

child has a facial disfigurement. They need reassurance, support and time to assimilate information. Having as accurate a diagnosis of the cleft as possible helps the family to visualise the child and to discuss feeding, especially breast feeding. It also helps discussion about the timing and type of surgery.

To plan appropriately for the future, parents need to discuss the management and likely treatment of the cleft at their own pace and in their own time, so that they are able to absorb this information. It is very important that, if parents wish to see pictures of clefts before and after surgery, they are shown pictures similar to the diagnosis of the cleft of their child. They also appreciate pictures which they can show to family and friends.

Parents normally imagine that their child will have a cleft similar to the worst

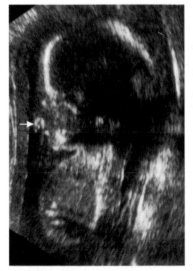

Scan 4.5.b: Prominence of pre-maxilla (arrowed): sagittal (lateral) plane

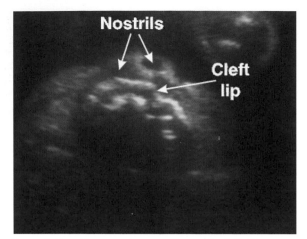

**Scan 4.5.c: Incomplete unilateral cleft lip:
Modified coronal plane**

pictures shown to them (Martin *et al*, Unpublished). It is not helpful to show a family expecting a child with a unilateral cleft, a picture of a bilateral one. During the pregnancy, some families appreciate a meeting with the surgeon and a visit to the ward where their baby will come for surgery. This helps them develop a strategy for coping with their child's need for an operation.

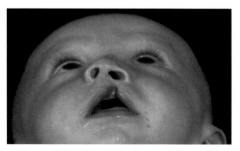

Figure 4.5c: Same baby as *Scan 4.5.c*

The support of lay people can be valuable for families diagnosed prenatally, but the choosing of families is difficult and should be done with extreme care (Turner and Milward, 1988). The family diagnosed prenatally should meet a family whose child has a similar cleft to their unborn child, so that the experiences shared are realistic. Parents who accept the role of looking after new families should either be vetted or perhaps even trained for the role that they undertake. Erwin and MacWilliams (1973) stressed that mothers with a problem were sometimes the most eager to become involved with others, even before they had resolved their own complicated feelings or developed any understanding about clefts in general. In these cases, there was a danger that the visiting mother may project her own difficulties into the new situation.

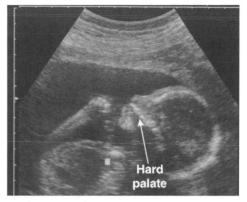

Scan 4.5.d: Normal hard palate: sagittal (lateral) plane

Prenatal diagnosis of a cleft lip is now commonplace. If parents are referred promptly to an experienced cleft team, they can be empowered with information and be better prepared for the birth. It is quite possible that, in spite of this information and support, some parents will opt to abort their child. The ethical issue of this is beyond the scope of this chapter.

While the prenatal diagnosis of facial clefting adds to the stress of pregnancy, it is our experience that when the child is born it invariably looks better than the parents envisaged. The anxiety, created by parents worrying about their child having the worst sort of cleft may be alleviated in the future by 3D scanning. This can give parents a more realistic picture of their child.

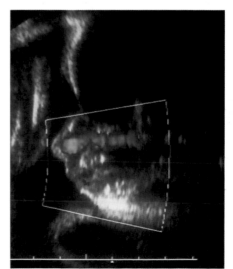

Scan 4.5.e: Colour flow doppler demonstrating intact hard palate

Parents who are unprepared for the birth of a child with a cleft lip often experience overwhelming shock and behave irrationally (Drotar,1975). To then care for the child when they are physically and mentally exhausted from the birth, is much more difficult. In contrast, parents whose child is diagnosed pre-natally, and are properly informed and supported, appear to enjoy giving birth and meeting their child for the first time. Parents appear better equipped to cope and the relationship between the child and the family appears happier and more secure.

The author's team arrange a meeting with the primary care team before the birth of the baby. This meeting is attended by the general practitioner, community and hospital midwife and health visitor who, with the parents and clinical nurse specialist from the cleft team, plan the initial management and care of the baby. More mothers appear able to breast feed or feed their baby with expressed breast milk as a result of this support.

5

Counselling

Patricia Bannister

Parents are the first significant people in a newborn infant's life, and the quality of that relationship is crucial in helping a child reach its physical and emotional potential. For an infant with a facial cleft, the importance of this role cannot be overemphasised, but parents will often need help to achieve this outcome. It is now generally accepted that adequate and accurate information is required and a plethora of resources exists to provide this, but services tend to concentrate on the infant, assuming that once parents are adequately informed the normal relationship will follow. Robertson (1962) states that the post natal period from birth to two months is one of adaptation, and successful adjustment has been achieved when a mother expresses pleasure in both her infant and her own mothering. Such an adapting period may be prolonged where there is a cleft, as the necessary changes in parenthood plans often interrupts this process. The aim of care and counselling is to ensure that adaptation is successful.

Society's collective beliefs about the significance of facial disfigurement varies considerably, and the support and subsequent coping behaviours used by individuals and families is, to a large extent, dependent on these values and expectations. Many myths exist as to the definition and importance of beauty, but they do have an immense impact on our thinking and actions (Changing Faces). Communities are now multi-cultural and it may be difficult for health professionals to understand and respond to the varying values, inherent in the different cultures. Nonetheless, parent's needs are now being recognised and nurses need to continue to explore ways in which these needs can be met.

The diagnosis of a cleft, either by ultrasound in the ante natal period, at birth or, in the post natal period, constitutes a traumatic event in parent's lives. Responses vary and the often painful process of adjusting to their imperfect baby is complicated and confused by the need to let go of the idealised perfect infant that they had anticipated (Solnit and Stark, 1962). During this period, responses are often described in terms of a bereavement. As in grief, parents experience varying degrees of shock, denial, anger, distress and anxiety (Kubler Ross, 1970). Others express feelings of inferiority at having produced or nurtured an imperfect child (Lax, 1972) and, if the baby is seen as an extension of the parent's own image, such emotions can have a powerful impact on parents vulnerable self esteem. Many parents express a feeling of loss of control that, despite their attempts at a healthy pregnancy, they have been unable to control the outcome. These parents often place great importance on their lives being under control and such a loss may lead to feelings of helplessness and depression (Seligman, 1975). Mothers especially may feel intense guilt as they feel their bodies are the custodians and nurturers of their unborn child. Questions as to what they should or should not have done during pregnancy are frequently asked. For many parents, as they gather resources, these intense feelings rapidly dissipate (Clifford and Crocker, 1971), but for others this adjustment is not so easy. All parents will need some help in making sense of these confused emotions.

Professional interventions

The attitudes of health professionals profoundly affect parents' emotions and behaviour in the immediate post partum and post natal period. Parents are particularly sensitive to the responses of others and are watching and evaluating the behaviour of doctors, nurses, midwives, and health visitors towards their baby. Any discomfort or anxiety displayed at this time will inevitably be transmitted to parents, and there is a need for health professionals to examine their own attitudes towards facial disfigurement and effectively evaluate them. Although at this time parents may be in shock, they are often immensely protective of their newborn infant, and any adverse rejection or comment from a nurse or doctor might result in parents rejecting future communication with that person. Nurses are often placed in a dual role of providing directive and non-directive care. In addition to practically caring for a mother following delivery, or a child following surgery, there is a need for simultaneous facilitative support and help. The fluid movement between these two roles in any one situation is difficult and inevitably directed by the assessment of need. Where a nurse frequently faces difficult situations, he/she needs to be aware of the dangers of reduplication and repetition (Winnicott, 1987), which sometimes leads to a hardening in her/his response to the parent and a prediction of their likely emotional response. 'I know how you feel' or 'don't worry', built on the experience gained from others is often unhelpful and belittles a parent's concerns. Avoidance of pessimism or unrealistic optimism is particularly important.

Winnicott (1987) states that, inevitably, such a condition carries with it an initial state of dependency, and what is required of the nurse is dependability and reliability. He speaks of the necessity for hierarchy to 'drop away', with parents and nurses meeting as equal human beings. There are many accounts of the prerequisites of a rich interpersonal relationship. In the role of carer/curer, there needs to be empathy, acceptance of parental reactions, a non judgmental approach, truthfulness and honesty, reliability and cross identification, the ability to stand in another person's shoes. The concept of 'holding' (Winnicott, 1987) provides a secure trusting relationship, enabling parents to personally grow. If these conditions are met, parents are more likely to move from a state of dependency to independency.

One of the most important counselling skills used by nurses is the skill of active listening. To listen and to concentrate on another person's conversation without introducing one's own thoughts, is often the least practised principle in human interactions. A nurse is often faced with the situation of two people with differing needs and anxieties. One parent may assume dominance in any conversation and it is important to establish both parents' anxieties before either are addressed. Some parents find talking disturbing and, while respecting this hesitancy in moving forward, it may be useful to bring other parents' feelings into the conversation to initiate discussion. A mother's dependency needs, first seen in pregnancy, continue to grow throughout the post partum period. She will need the support and acceptance of her family/partner and it is useful to establish if these relationships are normally communicative and open. Each family member will be experiencing their own grief and may not be aware of a mother's increased needs. An appreciation of the often difficult task for fathers of informing relatives of the bad news is a welcome approach, and begins to meet the needs of fathers.

Following the birth or after surgery, parents may not immediately feel able to care for their infant, and it is important for the nurse to be directly involved in exploring and touching the child with them, but not take away the responsibility of caretaking. Most infants with clefts are discharged home within the normal post partum period, but a few will require a prolonged stay. Mothers who are separated from their babies require increased sensitivity and encouragement to become involved with their infant. Mothers often express hesitation at interfering with the nurse who has assumed the caring role for their child and, as soon as permitted, need to be encouraged to participate in the normal activities of exploration, gazing, stroking, and cuddling. Although most special care units have protocols encouraging parent involvement, parents are often inhibited from initiating parent activities and are not always confident enough to control and organise their involvement. There is a need for specialist care and normal parenting activities to be separated, with clear boundaries delineating the responsibilities parents can assume.

Information

It is important that parents are given accurate and up-to-date information about their child's cleft. Information about other clefts is irrelevant, often confusing and increases unnecessary anxiety. Such information should be given in a language that is understandable and based upon any previous knowledge that parents may have about clefts and biological processes. It is important that the pace at which information is given is directed by the parents, as there is a danger that this process can come to resemble a tape recording of regurgitated facts. Such delivery is often a waste of time, in some cases causing parents to stop listening or misinterpret the facts. Accurate information, about normal anatomical and physiological processes, and the alterations that may have occurred, will undoubtedly increase parents' understanding of how they can manage their child. These are important prerequisites for decision-making and resumption of control as parents. Photographs and diagrams are important visual aids, but, before their use, it is important to identify what each parent would like to see. Many ante natal parents may not be ready to look at photographs of un-repaired clefts at diagnosis, but would be happy to see photographs of children following surgery.

In principle—good counselling/support

- **Antenatal preparation**. Discussion of termination should begin with parents and not be initiated by professionals

- The infant should be welcomed into the world in the same way as any other infant

- Parents require sensitive and empathetic support while exploring and examining their infant

- Parents should have early contact with a designated member of the cleft team

- Parents should be given time and encouragement to express their concerns and emotional response

- The needs of both parents must to be explored

- Parents should be given accurate information at a pace that is directed by them

- Nurses needs to examine their own beliefs and responses to facial disfigurement, and seek help or training, if there is any difficulty

- Nurses should approach each new family as a fresh encounter, unconditionally and honestly

- Parents should feel respected and cared for in terms of their needs; e.g. regaining control of their plans for their infant, availability of meals (especially if the mother appears unwilling to leave her infant)

- Communication between family members should be encouraged

- Initial dependency should be recognised, and the move to independency and normalisation of family life needs to be the long term goal.

Conclusion

The successful use of support and counselling skills are aimed at assisting parents to accept their child and form normal attachments. Although this adaptive period may last longer than normal, with skilled counselling it is achievable. Unresolved issues during these early years may affect or influence a parent's ability to counsel and support their growing child. Many parents are able to appreciate their own personal growth in this period and the part played by the nurse. For others, if things are going well, they take this for granted.

6
Feeding a baby with a cleft lip and palate

Introduction

Patricia Bannister

The successful feeding of any infant plays an integral part in the early mother/infant relationship. The feeding situation provides the initial forum for much of the early mother/infant interaction. If feeding is easy and satisfying, the mother will feel greatly encouraged and the feedback from her contented baby increases confidence in her ability to care for the newborn infant. If, in contrast, feeding is difficult and laborious, the mother feels inadequate as a parent and feelings of frustration and inadequacy may lead to her seeking alternative methods in an attempt to increase the likelihood of success and her own confidence. Parents must develop essential skills for breast/ bottle feeding. They enter parenthood with ideas of how they will feed their baby based, either on previous experience, or joint plans made with a partner, during the antenatal confinement. Modifications and adjustments are inevitable and it is important that families are given the necessary assistance to make these changes and assume their ordinary life styles. Some families are able to integrate these easily and require very little help; for others, however, the transition is more difficult. An increase in the understanding of family functioning has meant that the infant is no longer the singular focus of care.

Most infants with a cleft have early feeding problems only, but it is essential that these difficulties are dealt with in a way that does not lead to later cognitive, emotional, and functional difficulties for the child, which may affect eating patterns and growth. The main aims of feeding the infant with a cleft are the same as for any other infant, and all aspects of feeding need to be considered when planning care. Initial feeding assessment and planning, in the early neonatal period, should be seen as the foundation for the development of normal oral and cognitive development, and short term goals should not compromise the long term outcome. For babies with feeding difficulties, assessment and planning must be communicated to the primary care teams to ensure continued progress. This makes early and thorough discharge planning of the greatest importance.

Normal feeding

Full term healthy infants are born with the natural ability to feed and this oral activity is reflex driven. Stimulated through cranial nerve input, it is a co-ordinated way of receiving affective nutrition. Some of these reflexes remain for life, e.g. the gag reflex, while others are only utilised during early childhood and replaced by voluntary oral muscular activity (Ardveson, 1993). A baby seeks the nipple or teat by rooting and gaping and, on entering the mouth, the nipple stimulates a sucking reflex by coming into contact with the tongue and sensitive areas on the palate (Woolridge, 1986). Sucking activity results in the baby closing his/her lips around the teat/nipple and creating negative intra oral pressure. Anatomical differences equip the baby with an effective safety mechanism in the oro pharynx. The uvula and epiglottis lie adjacent, which means that fluid cannot enter the oro/hypo pharynx until the swallowing reflex is triggered. In the non cleft baby, milk is able pool in the baby's mouth safely until swallowing is triggered.

If sufficient negative intra oral pressure is created, the nipple is effectively placed for breast feeding (Woolridge, 1986) and, in bottle feeding, milk is delivered into the baby's mouth. The milk bolus is propelled backwards by the peristaltic movement of the tongue and triggers a swallow reflex. The soft palate elevates to occlude the naso pharynx and nasal breathing is suspended as milk moves into the pharynx. If there is insufficient intra oral pressure, the bolus of milk in the mouth is insufficient to trigger the swallow reflex and a change in sucking activity is noted.

Throughout any given feed, a baby demonstrates two sucking activities. These are known as non nutritive sucking and nutritive sucking (Brown, 1972). Non nutritive sucking is ineffective for successful feeding and is usually a result of a baby's inability to deliver milk into the mouth. Nutritive sucking is essential for effective feeding. The linkage of suck/swallow with nasal breathing can be achieved consistently only by infants of more than 37 weeks post conceptual age. Suck/swallow is established by 32 to 34 weeks gestation, but these babies are less effective at safe feeding and are unable to produce a one-to-one-to-one ratio of suck/swallow/breath (Bu Lock *et al*, 1990). There are many other anomalies and obstetric events that may interfere with the infant's ability to utilise effective and safe feeding during the early postpartum period.

Early considerations

Babies born with a cleft may present with a variety of feeding problems. The difficulties with an isolated cleft lip or cleft lip/palate can usually be resolved in early infancy, whereas infants born with an isolated cleft of the palate may take many months of careful assessment and management to achieve the same goal. This is particularly apparent in babies born with additional micrognathia or other syndromic conditions. Many studies have identified a wide range of problems, some of which are obvious at birth, while others only become evident with increasing age. Sometimes suspicions are aroused if the newborn exhibits an uncharacteristic feeding pattern. Studies have indicated that many of these babies fail to thrive in their early years (Seth and McWilliams, 1988), but it is the authors' opinion that, without effective assessment, planning and support from a specialist team, this is not always seen and more research is needed to support this.

Feeding breast milk to a baby with a cleft lip and palate

Vanessa Martin

The advantages of feeding a baby with a cleft lip and palate with breast milk cannot be over emphasised. The many benefits have been widely publicised, e.g. Unicef UK leaflet. Giving breast milk to a baby with a cleft lip and/or palate has added advantages:

- It is less irritating to the exposed and delicate tissue of the nose in babies with a cleft palate (babies having formula milk are inclined to produce more nasal secretions)

- It protects against nose and throat infections, which can contribute to the development of otitis media with effusion

- Breast milk acts as added protection for babies against infections when their resistance is low following their lip and palate operations

- Starving time can be reduced from approximately 5 hours to 2 hours when the baby is receiving breast milk (Phillips *et al*, 1994).

Many mothers have reported how valuable they have felt giving breast milk to their baby who has been born prematurely or with other anomalies.

Developing a feeding plan with the family

After pre-natal diagnosis of a baby with a cleft lip/palate and before the baby's birth is an ideal opportunity to discuss the parent's preferred feeding method. Even if the mother has already decided to feed her baby with formula milk, discussing the special qualities of colostrum is advantageous. The fact that low volumes of colostrum are high in nourishment, have anti-infective properties, and have a laxative effective, which helps clear meconium from the bowel, are some of the important factors that can be stressed. Skin to skin following the birth is important to discuss as this helps to calm the baby, keep him warm, steady his breathing and heart rate, and often leads naturally to his first breast feed. The routine of breast feeding and 'topping up' a baby with a cleft lip and palate is time-consuming, but mothers who have fed in this way feel a great sense of achievement. Mothers of twins, one of which has a cleft lip and palate, have opted to breast feed the twin without the cleft and expressed for the other twin, so that the father can bottle feed with expressed breast milk (EBM). This enables both parents to share in the feeding experience.

Babies with an isolated cleft lip

Babies with an isolated cleft lip are usually able to breast feed well, as the breast moulds into the cleft in the lip and helps to create the necessary seal for good attachment. Once the baby has learned to attach, he should have no difficulty in breast-feeding. Parents may wish to experiment with different positions, some preferring to feed with their baby positioned with the gap of the cleft down to occlude the gap with breast tissue, others preferring to use a finger in the gap to create a good seal. Babies with a wide unilateral cleft, which involves the lip and the alveolus, may need extra help in learning to attach.

Babies with a cleft lip and/or palate

Any baby who has a cleft which involves the palate will have abnormal placement of the soft palate muscles (see *Chapter 2: Figures 2.c and 2.d*). Because of this abnormal muscle position, there is limited and ineffective movement of the soft palate needed to create a vacuum in the mouth to draw in and to maintain the position of the breast for breast-feeding (Black *et al*, 1998). Some babies with a cleft lip and/or palate are much more difficult to breast feed successfully than others. These include:

- Babies with an extensive bilateral cleft lip and palate
- Babies with an isolated cleft that affects both hard and soft palate
- Babies with an isolated cleft palate, micrognathia and a tongue which is set back in the mouth

● Babies who have respiratory difficulties associated with their cleft palate.

Whether the cleft of the palate is small or large, initially, the baby will have difficulty in stimulating the supply of milk to maintain his volume requirements and a good weight gain. A mistake frequently made is that, because the baby is displaying rhythmical sucking movements at the breast, he is obtaining a nourishing milk supply. Even mothers with an abundant supply of milk may find their baby is not satisfied. They then tend to believe it is their inadequacy or the quality of their milk that is at fault, when it is the inability of the baby to remove the hind or fat-rich milk at the end of the feed, which causes the baby to be unsettled and to loose weight. For this reason, we recommend all mothers of babies with cleft palate to top up after each breast feed with expressed breast milk. Once baby's growth curve is established and the technique of latching on to the breast has improved, the amount of milk used to top up the baby following a breast feed can begin to be reduced.

Breast milk expression

It is helpful for a mother who wishes to breast feed, if she can begin to express her milk from 36 weeks. If the mother can be taught hand expression, this is the most efficient method of removing colostrum. Even the small amounts that are produced can be frozen, brought into hospital and given to the baby in addition to his first feed. If the mother is familiar with hand expression before the birth, she will find this easier than using the pump for milk removal for the first day or two. Hand expression for milk removal and electric pumping to stimulate the milk supply is recommended at first. Then, once the breast milk is beginning to establish, a portable electric double pump will be the most efficient method of milk expression. Double pumping can take as little as ten minutes to achieve breast emptying, and will ensure that the fat content in the expressed breast milk is higher (Jones *et al*, 2001). Ideally, the mother should be encouraged to express 6–8 times in 24 hours (not necessarily at regular intervals). This includes at least one expression during the night when prolactin levels are highest. It does help to have at least one feed ahead for the baby. If the mother can have her own breast pump, she will be more likely to achieve a good production of milk. She should be encouraged when using the pump to start the vacuum low and, if she wishes, to increase the pressure once the milk starts to flow. The breast shield should be applied with enough pressure to produce a vacuum, but not too much pressure so that the flow is reduced. Using the pump at her baby's feed time and when he/she is close will help to increase the flow.

For mothers whose baby is in the neo-natal unit, having a picture of their baby with them may help when they are expressing. Once the flow of milk is established, the mother may need to spend more time using the breast pump to ensure that all the milk has been removed. Complete milk removal will secure a plentiful supply for the future. Any excess can be stored in the freezer and used by the baby-sitter if the mother wishes to have an evening out, or even saved for the baby's hospital admission.

Calculating baby's feed

If the baby is having expressed breast milk by bottle or by naso-gastric tube, a rough guide on calculating the amount of feed he/she requires from day five onwards is as follows:

Baby's weight in kilos is multiplied by 150mls and divided by the number of feeds in 24 hours

For example, a 3kg weight x 150mls = 450mls in 24 hours. 450 ÷ 8 (for 3 hourly feeds) = 56mls per feed and 450 ÷ 6 (for 4 hourly feeds) = 75mls per feed.

This is a rough guide only. Babies require less feed during the first five days and, if they have been born prematurely, may be discharged home on a higher volume per kilogram.

For babies who are attaching to the breast and breast feeding, it is recommended that those with cleft palate involvement are offered at least three quarters of their requirement as a top up, or whatever amount the mother can can produce, until the child appears satisfied.

Breast feeding

Breast-feeding is both rewarding and satisfying, but those mothers who have difficulty in getting their child to attach to the breast, and who opt to express their milk and give it by bottle, often feel that this is second best for their baby. This is not so. The dedication required to express milk and give this expressed milk to their child is to be admired, and mothers should be proud to have achieved this, even for a short period.

The technique of breast feeding

Breast-feeding has been achieved most successfully long term, by parents of babies with cleft palate involvement, who have been taught an exaggerated attachment technique.

To achieve this technique, the baby should be correctly positioned with his body in a straight line facing the mother and his nose opposite his mother's nipple. The mother's hand should support the breast underneath with her small finger touching her ribs. Her thumb should rest on the top of the breast, usually on the edge of the areola and baby's nose should be in line with the nipple, so that he can smell the milk and open his mouth wide. Baby's bottom lip should make contact with the areola well away from the base of the nipple. The nipple should then be tilted with the mother's thumb, so that the baby opens his mouth as wide as possible.

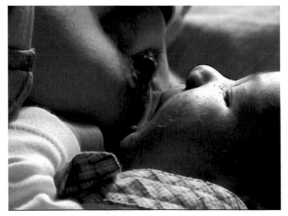

Figure 6.1: Latching on (1)

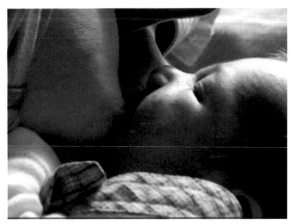

Figure 6.2: Rolling the nipple

The thumb should then be used to quickly slide or role the nipple forward under the roof of the baby's mouth, (see leaflets by Unicef UK; and Martin and Abbett, 2003).

If the baby can take as much breast as possible into his mouth, he will stay attached to the breast for a longer period of time. It may be necessary to help him to maintain this breast hold by the mother keeping her thumb and finger in the stabilising position.

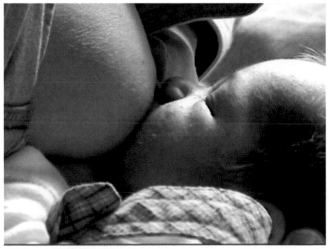

Figure 6.3: Latched on (4)

Figures 6.4.a/b/c: Exaggerated attachment technique

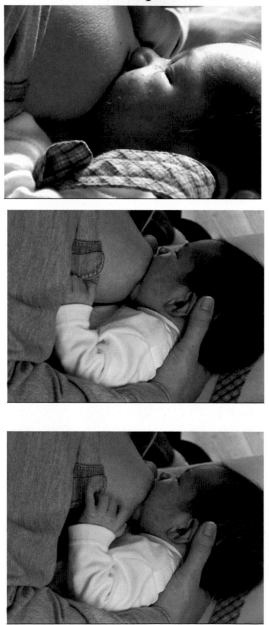

A baby who is well attached will obtain milk more easily. Babies who do well in spite of poor attachment do so because the mother has an abundance of milk. Problems with milk flow can be overcome if the mother is taught breast compression. This may also result in her baby taking more of the milk that is high in fat. Breast compression is achieved by the mother holding the breast with her thumb on one side and fingers on the other, fairly far back from the nipple. As the baby is drinking, the mother compresses the breast, keeping up the pressure to increase milk flow (Newman, 2000). Encouraging the mother to snuggle her baby and skin-to-skin contact occasionally without feeding will help her milk production.

Breast feeding and topping up

If the baby has a cleft of the palate, it is important that he is topped up after each feed with expressed breast milk until he has established a good breast feeding technique, or his weight is established on a centile curve. Expressed breast milk is usually given given after each breast-feed. This 'topping up' is important, as research has shown that initial weight gain is slower in some babies with a cleft palate (Avedian and Ruberg, 1980; Brine *et al*, 1994; Jones, 1988). Many cleft babies in Nepal and probably other developing countries have difficulty maintaining their weight on breast feeding alone (Martin, 1999).

Sometimes, if a baby is offered a bottle and teat while establishing breast-feeding, he may become confused when put to the breast. This is because, when breast feeding:

- A different feeding style if required

- A wider opening of the mouth is needed to accommodate the nipple

- A stronger tongue action is needed to stimulate the milk.

For this reason, when the baby is first 'topped up', it is usually recommended that this top up feed is offered by cup or a bottle with a scoop.

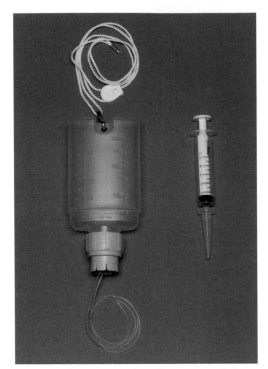

Figure 6.5: Supplementary Nursing System and finger feeder

There are also devices that can help deliver extra milk during the breast feed, for example, a Lactaid or Supplementary Nursing System (SNS Central Medical Supplies), a bottle that mother can hang around her neck and which delivers expressed breast milk, while the baby is attached to her breast), or a finger feeder used in conjunction with a syringe (see *Figure 6.5*). This can also be affective in assisting infants to latch on to the breast. A video on its use is available (Herzog/Isler, 1994).

The specialist nurse from the cleft team may be able to advise on these methods of feeding. Individual plans of breast feeding, topping up and expressing should be reviewed periodically. If the mother is able to produce adequate supplies of milk, expressing may gradually be reduced from 6–8 times a day, although this may reduce the mother's milk production. Indications that the baby is getting enough breast milk are that he should have at least 6–8 wet nappies a day and his bowel action should be bright yellow.

Expressing your milk while baby is in hospital

Unless the children's ward has its own breast pump, mothers should be advised to take their own pumps into hospital with them when the baby has the operation. This is a stressful time and it is easy to forget it. Initially, on admission, the mother can follow her normal routine of breast feeding/expressing. The baby will not be allowed to feed for at least three hours before the operation, if he is having breast milk. Once he stops breast feeding or having expressed breast milk, the mother should be encourage to express at least four hourly, depending on her supply of milk. Once the baby is re-established on breast feeding/expressed breast milk, it is still advisable to decrease the expressing gradually until the child is re-established on full feeds (adapted from Martin and Abbett, 2003).

Bottle feeding

Patricia Bannister

Cleft lip and palate

Feeding difficulties related to the full term baby with an isolated cleft of the lip and those involving the lip and palate are generally related to reduced sucking efficiency. The baby is unable to produce sufficient negative intra oral pressure due to the anatomical defects in the cleft lip and/or palate. Reflex activity in most incidences is normal. It is important, during the first 48 hours following delivery, that a baby is allowed time to safely organise suck/swallow/breath co-ordination. A cleft palate removes that safety barrier between the mouth, naso pharynx, and oro pharynx making it difficult for the baby to contain the bolus of milk in the mouth prior to swallow. Aggressive feeding at this stage is not advised.

For mothers who choose to bottle feed their infants, safety is maintained by using a normal unadjusted teat and hard bottle for the first few feeds and any particular difficulty noted prior to the more detailed feeding assessment. For the baby with an isolated cleft lip, minor adjustments to the teat may be all that is necessary, as sucking inefficiency is very small. Where there is a cleft involving the lip, alveolus and palate, whether unilateral or bilateral, a more pronounced sucking inefficiency is observed and the baby will require teat adjustments and 'assisted feeding' (Shaw *et al*, 1999) using a soft plastic bottle. Effective nutritive suckling is important to negate the possibility of lengthy feeds, ingestion of large amounts of air, and fatigue.

Babies demonstrate two distinct patterns of sucking and both are observable during an oral feed. The principle difference is the effective delivery of milk into the mouth for swallowing. Non-nutritive sucking is best observed when an infant is sucking on a dummy, sucking on a teat, but unable to remove the milk from the bottle, or when a baby is first put to the breast and is gently stimulating the let down reflex of milk. It occurs in short, sharp bursts at a rate of two per second and there is very little forward thrust, forward movement of the mandible. Rhythmical non-nutritive sucking is a necessary skill for oral feeding and may be observed in the premature infant from about thirty weeks gestation, or in the baby who has difficulty in swallowing (dysphagia). Nutritive sucking occurs at a slow rate of one per second, and a more pronounced forward movement of the mandible is observed, effectively placing milk on the tongue for swallowing. Patent nasal airways are essential for the successful development of both types of sucking activity. Nutritive sucking is organised and co-ordinated into a pattern of ten to fifteen suck/swallow/breath, followed by a short pause. Some infants are unable to achieve this pattern immediately and may be more comfortable with a combination of nutritive and non-nutritive sucks within a single burst.

In the early neonatal period, it may be difficult for the baby to stabilise the nipple or teat in the mouth, as the opposing palatal tissue surface is absent and the tongue may not have acquired the trough-like shape necessary to stabilise the teat. It is important that the feeder holds the nipple/teat firmly into the mouth, avoiding the 'jiggling movement' often adopted to promote sucking activity. Such activity may result in ulceration of the nasal septum or nasal turbinates, both of which may cause pain and distress.

Feeding position

For these babies there is no indication to nurse in any other position than that of the normal infant.

Isolated cleft palate

It is now understood that babies who are diagnosed with an isolated cleft palate require different management from those born with clefts involving the lip and/or palate (Shaw *et al*, 1999). They often produce a more complex feeding problem that, in many cases, cannot be resolved in the early post partum period. In addition to the anatomical defect, physiological alterations in the function of the tongue and oral pharynx contribute to these difficulties. A percentage of these babies are likely to have associated anomalies in which cleft palate is only one of the characteristics. The most common problem associated with cleft palate is varying degrees of micrognathia (small mandible), which often resolves spontaneously, (*Figure 6.b.c.d. and e*) and glossoptosis (retro placement of the tongue). These have a marked effect on the baby's ability to feed. It is perhaps useful to consider these babies on a continuum with those mildly affected at

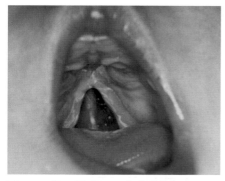

Figure 6.a: Palate of child on Page 60

one end and those more severely at the other extreme (Bannister, 2001). Minor feeding problems with the former are easily resolved with assisted feeding. For those infants more severely affected, Pierre Robin sequence, marked micro- gnathia and glossoptosis place the baby at high risk of respiratory obstruction, and a paediatric/anaesthetic assessment of airway stability is essential prior to any attempt at oral feeds. Marked tracheal tugging, sometimes accompanied by sternal or intercostal recession when the baby is supine, are early indicators of respiratory difficulties. A baby who is struggling

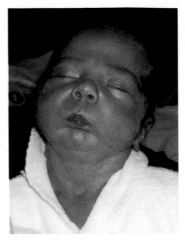

Figure 6.b: Severe micrognathia

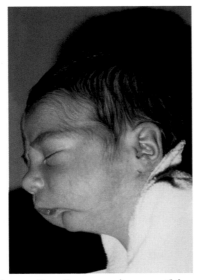

Figure 6.c: Severe micrognathia

to maintain an adequate airway is at high risk of aspiration if orally fed (Bath and Bull, 1997; Shprintzen, 1988).

A baby's position on the continuum is not always stable and, following the introduction of oral feeding, it is advisable to continue to assess respiratory stability through observation and the regular assessment of blood gases. Babies may require the support of nasogastric tube feeding to prevent this deterioration. This may only be necessary for a few days, but, where it is indicated, usually continues for the first three to four months until the baby has grown and developed sufficient oro-muscular control to keep the tongue forward.

If nasogastric feeding is implicated, it is important to involve the parents from an early age so that they are able to adapt to their child's different needs as soon as possible. Non nutritive sucking, using a dummy at feeds times, will assist the

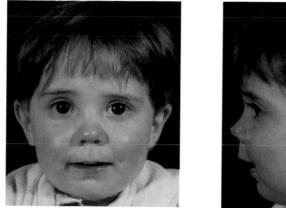
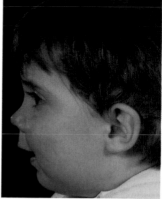

Figures 6.d and e: Catch up growth of chin with age (3 years)

continued development of oral skills and enhance the growth in the cognitive link between sucking and satiation of hunger.

Once teat feeding has commenced, careful assessment and planning is required as to the frequency and length of time an infant is allowed to oral feed, so as to maintain airway stability. It is important that baby's experience of feeding is a pleasant one. Joint planning with the clinical nurse specialist on the cleft team is essential.

Position for babies with respiratory problems

For these infants, feeding in the normal cradling position is often dangerous. Infants are safer and more comfortable nursed prone or on their sides. This is contrary to the supine position advised in the prevention of cot death, but an assessment of risks is important in the discussion. Oral feeding can successfully commence in the lateral position and the cradling position can only be considered when all evidence of respiratory symptoms have disappeared.

Other issues

Babies born with an isolated cleft palate often demonstrate increased calorific needs because of the increase in respiratory effort. Sometimes these can be met by increasing the feed to 180mls per kilo, adding a calorie supplement to normal volumes or, in particularly difficult social circumstances, prescribing a higher calorie milk. If combined with a reflux problem, the latter two suggestions are useful considerations when attempting to reduce volume without compromising calorie intake.

For other reflux difficulties, the use of antacids or specialized formula needs to be tried before other procedures or prescribed drugs are considered.

Feeding plates, once considered important, are now infrequently used. If correctly made, they seem to have a limited use in breast feeding (Herzog-Isler and Honigmann, 1996), but the author has not substantiated this.

Feeding assessment

Important factors in feeding assessment:

- Family, medical/social history
- Presence of other anomalies
- Obstetric history of baby's birth and gestational age
- Examination of head and face
- Presence of oral reflexes
- Co-ordination of skills
- Identification of the abilities and difficulties presented by the baby
- Parental teaching
- Identification of difficulties that can be resolved quite easily, and those requiring time and maturation
- Provision of plan and consistent feeding equipment including the loan of a breast pump if expressing milk

- Plans for discharge.

Principles of good management are:

- Sensitive and empathetic handling at delivery
- Nursing/paediatric assessment as to the extent of the anomalies and immediate management
- Early exploration of parental plans for feeding
- Breast and bottle feeding if appropriate on the labour ward
- Transfer of the mother and baby together, if appropriate, to the situation of their choice
- *Separation of mother from baby only when one or other requires medical intervention*
- Referral to the cleft team using agreed protocol
- Telephone cleft team for early advice
- Early feeding established using normal teat, bottle or breast
- *Appropriate methods of nutrition where oral feeding is not advised*
- Appropriate positioning of infant
- Allowing time with parents to listen to main anxieties and feelings
- Feeding assessment and feeding plan within the first 24 to 48 hours by a feeding specialist from the cleft team
- Short and long term aims and goals
- *If in special care, availability of parents for any oral feeding; otherwise, restriction in the number of carers so as to avoid confusion for the baby*
- Discharge planning
- Liaison with primary care team.

Assisted feeding

Difficulties related to insufficient negative intra-oral pressure can be made easier by enlarging the existing hole in the latex teat, making an additional hole using a red hot intramuscular needle or combining an adjusted/unadjusted teat with a soft flexible bottle. The bottle can be gently squeezed as the infant suckles, either in a continuous or pulse squeeze action. The ratio of suck to squeeze is decided following feeding assessment and it is dependent on the swallowing capability of the infant. Flexible bottles cannot be used safely when swallowing difficulties have been identified. Assistance may vary throughout a given feed or from one feed to the next, and parental teaching is important in order to maintain safe feeding. It is important to avoid distress and the nasal regurgitation of milk. The correct flow of milk promotes a relaxed baby with no nasal regurgitation, the development of good nutritive skills, and enhances oral development.

Feeding equipment

A study into feeding methods revealed that parents would prefer equipment that was as close to normal as possible (Shaw *et al*, 1999) and standardised teats and bottles are now available through the mail order service provided by the Cleft Lip and Palate Association (CLAPA).

- A commonly used teat is the NUK, size 2, orthodontic shaped latex teat. Latex teats are easily and safely adapted and can be combined with a soft bottle. The larger size teats span the cleft and are tolerated by neonates with a birth weight about 2.5kgs

- A NUK cleft palate teat is not always aesthetically acceptable and was found by Choi *et al* in 1991 not to generate negative intraoral pressure

- **Haberman feeding system**: This feeding system is used as an alternative to the soft bottle for assisted feeding. It is expensive and the shape of the teat can results in ulceration of the nasal turbulence. Because of its adjustable flow system, modification of the teat is unnecessary

- **Soft flexible bottle**: The Mead Johnson bottle is particularly useful for parents with problems involving their hands, e.g., arthritis or carpel tunnel. However, it is often

too soft and pliable for other parents. Other soft bottles, e.g.
Soft Plas, have sufficient pliability and have a regular bottle
shape (see *Figure 6.6*).

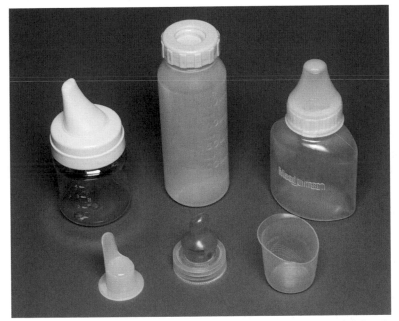

**Figure 6.6: From left to right: Top row—Spout for use with beaker
or bottle; Soft Plas bottle; Mead Johnson bottle
Bottom row—Scoop for use with Soft Plas bottle; NUK
orthodontic teat; Cup for early feeding**

Oral hygiene

For the first two to three months, babies produce very little
saliva. Where there is a cleft of the palate, this is often
insufficient to keep the oral and nasal passages clean. Two to
three teaspoons of cooled boiled water given after formula feeds
will reduce the likelihood of infection and 'snuffly' behaviour
often associated with formula feeding. This may be
discontinued with the maturational increase in saliva
production. Additional water is unnecessary when the baby is
receiving breast milk. The application of an edible lubricant,
either Vaseline or a nipple cream, to the area surrounding the
cleft lip and alveolus will help prevent soreness. The use of

cotton wool buds to clear inside the nose and mouth is not advisable, although their use may be helpful in removing debris from around the alar rim. Ulceration of the nasal septum is not uncommon and is usually not painful; it usually resolves within a few weeks. It is important to keep the teat still in the baby's mouth in order to help avoid damage. Ulceration of the nasal turbinates, however, is extremely painful and oral feeds with a teat may be difficult. Feeding using a scoop is acceptable for a few days to allow the area to heal.

Weaning

The COMA Report (1994) recommends that weaning foods should not be given to infants before the age of four months and that a mixed diet should be established by the age of six months. It is important that infants born with a cleft follow these guidelines and feeding difficulties, which may lead to early weaning, be addressed effectively. At about four months developmental age, an increase in the size of the mouth in relation to the tongue, and neurological maturation allows the baby to produce pre chewing skills (Schechter, 1990) in addition to suckling activity. This allows the infant to control pureed feed without nasal regurgitation. As the infant acquires this new skill, it may be helpful to introduce weaning foods half way through a milk feed and sit the baby in a chair. Using a soft spoon, rest the spoon on the tongue and lower lip while the baby removes the food from the spoon at his/her own pace. The transition to thicker, pureed, mashed and lumpy foods generally occurs at a similar age to any other infant and is not dependent on the closure of the palate. It is important not to miss these windows of developmental opportunity, but many parents require support in this transition as there are fears that food will become lodged in the cleft. There are various ways to build confidence, one of which is to offer taste of mashed foods at family meal times.

Removal of naso-gastric tube

The prolonged use of a naso-gastric (NG) tube after the immediate neo-natal period is usually confined to those babies with associated Pierre Robin Sequence or babies with additional anomalies, which may physically or neurologically affect oral feeding. With increasing age, growth and oro-motor development, by three to four months of age, these difficulties are usually beginning to resolve and the baby is able to integrate reflex skills with oro-motor skills. As this occurs, there are several ways to reduce the dependency on NG feeding but, in order for parents to achieve this, they will require a great deal of support and advice.

Some infants may gradually increase the amount that they are able to take from a teat and bottle and thus reduce the amount of supplementary feed. For others, however, parents and professionals need to recognise the baby's increased abilities and withdraw NG feeding to encourage the him/her to gain confidence in his/her own abilities. As weaning foods are increased, a baby is less dependant on a fluid diet and the calorie content of milk can be temporarily increased to maintain an adequate nutrition. Alternatively, NG feeds can be reduced to once daily, usually in the evening to maintain day/night feeding patterns. It may take several weeks for a baby to relinquish a dependency on the tube, but with patience and gentle persuasion this can, in most cases, be successfully achieved. Daily contact with parents, by telephone or home visit, is important in maintaining parental confidence.

The move to gastrostomy feeding must only be considered where marked neuro-muscular difficulties persist beyond this age, or when there are additional physical problems, such as pronounced cardiac anomalies. In all but a very small number of infants, this is unnecessary.

A successful transition can be measured in terms of adequate growth and a baby and parent who have a positive behavioural approach to eating and appetite.

Conclusion

Feeding is an important part of cleft care, but advice must be based on a sound understanding of normal feeding behaviours. Babies with a cleft of the lip, with or without palate involvement, need different management to those babies born with a isolated cleft palate. The development of a good feeding pattern should be based on long term goals not short term gains, and collaborative working with cleft lip and palate teams is essential. The successful teaching of good feeding behaviour is perhaps one of the most challenging aspects for nurses caring for these infants and their families.

With the reorganisation of cleft care in the United Kingdom, all district general hospitals should be linked to a regional cleft centre and the appropriate arrangements for early referral set in place (see *Chapter 1*). Guidelines state that once informed, a designated member of the cleft team is responsible for visiting the family within 24–48 hours following diagnosis. This allows a feeding assessment to be carried out as early as possible and prevents the development of harmful feeding patterns. A feeding plan can be made in conjunction with the parents, midwives and paediatric staff so that consistency of care is achieved.

7
ENT and related audiology

Vanessa Martin

A good speech outcome for children with a cleft palate depends primarily on two requirements: a functional repair of the palatal muscles and the ability to hear clearly. It is important that a child has good hearing to acquire good speech, since speech is developed through mimicking.

The association between a cleft of the palate and otitis media with effusion (glue ear) is well recognised. The main function of the eustachian tube is to ventilate the middle ear. The secondary function is to allow tiny amounts of mucus secreted to escape into the nasal pharynx. As the tensor palati muscle is mis-aligned in the child with a cleft palate, this can affect the function of the eustachian tube. It is suggested that eustachian tube dysfunction and defective ventilation of the middle ear changes the pathology of the middle ear mucosa, resulting in 'hyperplasia of the mucous glands' (Cowan and Kerr, 1986). This results in a sterile fluid accumulating in the middle ear causing a conductive hearing loss. This loss may be as little as 10 dB (decibels) or as much as 40 dB (Lennox, 2001), but is as if a child is hearing with his fingers in his ears. It may not only affect speech, but also behaviour and the ability to concentrate at school.

Other causes of eustachian tube dysfunction are inflammation of the mucosa of the nasopharynx caused by infection or allergy, and hypertrophy of the adenoids. There has been a suggestion that babies who are breast-fed are less likely to acquire the symptoms of otitis media (Paradise *et al*, 1994). It is certainly a known fact that breast-feeding reduces the risk of infections and allergy.

Management of otitis media with effusion (OME)

All specialist centres treating children with a cleft lip and palate should have a lead ENT surgeon responsible for the assessment and management of children with hearing loss. A protocol of care should be developed in each region, whereby each child with a cleft palate has his hearing assessed regularly. Otoacoustic emissions tests, which will be nationally available, can be performed on newborns to assess cochlea function, if middle ear function is normal. A negative test does not indicate the nature or severity of hearing loss, but that further testing is required. A more sophisticated auditory brain stem response test will confirm whether the hearing loss is conductive, or sensorineural requiring the child to be fitted with a hearing aid.

At this stage, a conductive hearing loss is unlikely to require treatment, although a repeat test is often recommended in three months. Some ENT surgeons will consider fitting grommets when cleft palate surgery is performed. Others wait and retest after the surgery to realign the tensor palati muscles, as this may improve the eustachian tube function. No research has, as yet, confirmed a correct management protocol.

When the child has sufficient head control, distraction tests can be performed. These are where an adult distracts the child and his response to sounds is observed. Later, pure tone audiometry, which assesses the volumes a patient can hear using an audiometer, or tympanometery, which measures the efficiency of the transmission of sound waves through the ear, can be used to assess a child's hearing.

Treatment

Persistent otitis media with effusion may require treatment involving a myringotomy and insertion of grommets. This is done under a general anaesthetic in a morning or afternoon's admission to hospital. The surgeon makes an incision in the tympanic membrane of the ear and removes the fluid by suction. He then inserts a grommet (ventilation tube), which replaces the function of the eustachian tube. Short-term grommets, such as Sheppard and Reuter grommets, are likely to remain in position for 6–9 months. T tubes and Per-lee grommets may stay in position indefinitely. The latter are often used in children with otitis media with effusion related to a cleft palate.

The insertion of grommets remains controversial. Damage to the tympanic membrane has been sighted as a reason for not inserting grommets (Robson *et al*, 1992) and timing of surgery is debated by others. Some surgeons will insert grommets routinely during cleft palate surgery, some when the hearing loss is persistent or substantial, and others if there are problems with speech. It is well recognised that persistent otitis media with effusion exacerbates speech and learning problems. These reasons (and related behavioural problems) are good indications of the need to treat glue ear.

8
Cleft lip and palate surgery

Mark Henley

The surgery of cleft lip and palate has evolved over the last century with the greatest changes over the last 50 years. Perhaps the greatest change has been the increasing acceptance that no one method, individual surgeon or philosophy provides the perfect solution, and that the only way in which results may be improved is by meaningful audit and prospective study. There has been an evolution of surgical procedures and I will deal with these by anatomical site.

Unilateral lip and nose

The lip repair of Ambrose Parre consisted of what was effectively a simple adhesion procedure with freshening of the margins of the cleft lip and suturing the margins together. This was commonly practised until about fifty years ago when individual surgeons attempted to restore a more normal anatomical appearance to the lip by the use of plastic surgical principles. There were many individual variations, but the three most popular in the UK were the 'Le Meseurier' with square flaps, the 'Tennison' with Z-plasties and the 'Millard' with rotation/advancement flaps. All these procedures involved the drawing of a pattern and then making incisions to match, with no attempt to correct the underlying abnormalities of orientation of muscle or cartilage. In Austria, Anderl developed a radical approach that involved freeing of all the abnormally located tissues and restoring normal anatomy and, in France, Delaire developed a 'functional' repair that particularly focussed upon the restoration of normal muscle anatomy. Marsh developed the concept of early adhesion and nasal correction. This relied upon the adhesion pulling the alveolar segments (gums) into line, effectively making the cleft incomplete. Desai explored neonatal repair, exploiting the malleability of the skull and facial bones in the neonate.

Most authorities (other than Anderl) regarded the nose as being a prohibited area at the time of primary repair, until the work of McComb and Piggott who demonstrated the benefits of early nasal correction and the absence of significant complications. Anderl had been practising primary nasal correction for many years with good results, but was not published widely in the English literature.

Current practice reflects these influences, with variation in both the timing and nature of the lip repair. Surgery may be undertaken at any time during the first six months of life depending upon the nature of the cleft and the surgical team.

The author treats wide unilateral clefts by neonatal adhesion, and primary nasal correction with definitive repair, six months after the initial procedure. He repairs incomplete clefts at around six months of age.

Bilateral cleft lip

The practice in respect of bilateral cleft lip is less well defined. It is generally accepted that this is a worse problem than unilateral clefts because there is an absence of muscle in the prolabial segment, and a degree of maxillary hypoplasia is inevitable. The alternatives of approach consist of alternatives of staged repair. One approach in current practice is to repair the widest side followed by the second as two unilateral lip repairs, a few weeks apart. The alternative is to perform a single stage repair of both sides, accepting that a second stage repair may be required at or around four to five years of age. More recently, Cutting and others have advocated a radical repair of the nose and lip with staged surgery to produce a nose appropriate for the age of the patient.

The author performs a single stage closure of the lip with a limited nasal correction. Although there is the possibility of a second stage being required, this does not appear to be inevitable. It is too early to say whether this offers any definite advantage over the established techniques and needs to be confirmed by long-term study.

Palate

Historically, palate repair was undertaken using palatal flaps. Depending upon the background of the surgeon concerned, the surgery was either restricted to the minimum possible to achieve repair, such as incision of the margins of the cleft and closure in layers, or a standard procedure was undertaken regardless of the nature of the cleft. 'Standard' procedures in the UK were principally the Von Langenbeck repair, with the use of lateral releasing incisions, or the Veau Wardill Kilner 'pushback', with the use of V-Y incisions in the anterior palatal mucoperiosteum. These procedures were typically undertaken between 14 and 18 months of age. Alternatives practised in Europe involved repair of the soft palate at any time between three and six months, and secondary repair of the hard palate, generally between one and three years later, although Schweckendeck delayed this until eight years.

Furlow introduced the use of Z-Plasties to effect repair of the levator muscle sling and closure of the soft palate, and this was popularised by Randall and others. It remains popular in global practice.

Sommerlad developed the concept of undertaking radical intravelar veloplasty and levator sling reconstruction with the assistance of the operating microscope.

The Eurocleft study demonstrated a need for more structured study and audit of surgical techniques and, although not yet fully established, surgical practice in the UK is evolving in this direction.

Again, the current surgical practice reflects the nature of the cleft and the training of the surgeon.

The author repairs isolated clefts of the palate at around six months in the manner described by Sommerlad, with limited releasing incisions where required.

Submucous clefts of the palate are notorious. The relative lack of success using standard techniques meant that, for many surgeons, the treatment of choice was a primary pharyngoplasty. Sommerlad reported reasonable success using a radical intravelar veloplasty and in Nottingham this type of cleft is repaired using his technique. However, following the work of Milward, the Furlow technique is considered by many to be more reliable.

Complete clefts of the hard and soft palate and those occurring in combination with clefts of the lip are repaired either in combination with the definitive lip repair, or in a staged manner with repair of the soft palate and delayed repair of the hard palate at one year following, the approach developed by the Gothenburg unit. Lateral releasing incisions are utilised where it is considered appropriate to effect closure at one stage.

Secondary surgery of the palate

Secondary surgery of the palate is undertaken for velopharyngeal incompetence (VPI). This section will focus on the management of VPI related to cleft palate, although it must be recognised that the most common cause is neurological and such cases can only rarely be managed in the manner described below.

Historically, the management of this problem varied considerably according to the surgeon and support facilities available. Treatment varied from neglect—the author is aware of at least one case where an otherwise normal person was admitted to an asylum because of their speech defect and who became totally institutionalised and incapable of independent existence. Patients were treated conservatively with tuition in accommodating their speech and passive plates to occlude fistulae and support the soft palate. Assessment prior to surgery was very variable and the definition of significant VPI warranting surgery remains ill defined. Extremes vary from misting of a mirror placed beneath the nostrils during speech, to total lack of intelligibility. The decision to operate was generally that of the surgeon alone, with very variable input from other specialists and, particularly, speech therapists.

The surgery was generally that which the surgeon had learned or felt most comfortable with, and reduction of the size of the velopharyngeal port was achieved by one of three types of procedure: a sphincter pharyngoplasty, construction of a flap between the posterior pharyngeal wall and the soft palate, or augmentation of the posterior wall of the pharynx.

Over the last fifteen to twenty years, there has been significant change in the management of VPI, and much of the credit for this must go to Piggott and Sommerlad.

Piggott advanced the investigation of palatal movement with combined lateral videofluouroscopy and nasendoscopy. He proposed the concept of tailoring the surgery to address the functional defect. Sommerlad developed the concept of palate rerepair. He used an operating microscope to define the surgical anatomy in much greater detail than was previously possible and, following on from his work, others have developed the use of the Furlow 'Z-Plasty' to undertake rerepair.

Boorman and colleagues have recently reported a predictor based upon the degree of velar closure on lateral videofluouroscopy, which can be used to decide whether to consider rerepair or proceed direct to pharyngoplasty.

More recently, Sell and Mars at Great Ormond Street have further developed the use of speech bulbs to provide passive closure of isolated lateral defects, or where muscle function is poor.

Some success with augmentation of the posterior pharyngeal wall using Teflon has been reported from the United States when the defect was 6mm or less, but others have reported sleep apnoea as a complication. Anecdotal reports suggest that the South African experience using costal cartilage grafts has been encouraging. At present, the use of endoscopic assisted surgery is under development, and it is hoped that this will also contribute to the success rate by permitting better visualisation and greater precision of surgery.

Procedures for velopharyngeal incompetence

Palate re-repair (Sommerlad)

This is the simplest of the secondary procedures and is suitable for cases where there is good muscle function, but a persistent small defect in closure of the velopharyngeal port. At nasendoscopy, such cases will show as a 'v' shape of the soft palate instead of the normal dome (*Figure 8.i*). This indicates tethering of the palatal muscles, generally by scar tissue to the

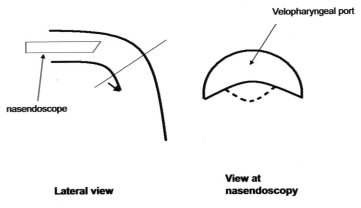

Velopharyngeal port

nasendoscope

Lateral view

View at nasendoscopy

Figure 8.1: The soft palate

back of the hard palate. The operation consists of dissecting the muscles and scar tissue free from the bone and reconstructing the levator muscle sling as far back as possible (*Figure 8.2*). The dissection is facilitated by the use of the operating microscope. The advantages are that recovery is rapid and there are few complications or long term sequelae. The anatomy is restored to

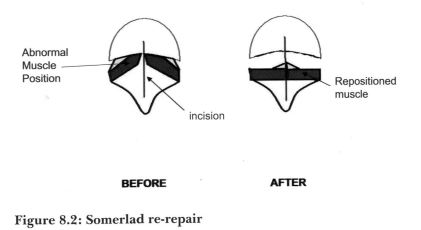

Abnormal Muscle Position

incision

Repositioned muscle

BEFORE

AFTER

Figure 8.2: Somerlad re-repair

as near normal as possible and, in the event that the procedure does not produce a wholly successful outcome, no other surgical options have been lost. The limitations are that the procedure is only suitable for selected cases where the defect is small and the underlying muscle function is good. In addition, the surgical scar is straight and in the midline so any scar contracture will have a tethering effect on the soft palate. Audit has demonstrated that this procedure produces best results in patients under the age of 10 years

Furlow procedure *(Figure 8.3)*

The Furlow procedure uses Z-Plasties to effect reconstruction of the levator sling and lengthening of the soft palate, and is widely used for primary repair. The procedure requires dissection, which is more limited and less precise than the Sommerlad rerepair. This can be a significant advantage when dealing with very scarred tissues. The transposition of the flaps produces physical lengthening of the soft palate and the zig zag nature of the scars means that any natural scar contracture will tend to produce lengthening rather than tethering. As with the

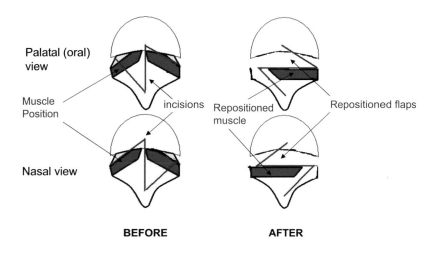

Figure 8.3: Furlow re-repair

rerepair, the limitations are: that there must be good underlying muscle function, and the defect should be small to moderate in size. Anatomy of the muscles is restored to normality, but the mucosa is not and any further palatal surgery must take account of the potential risk to the blood supply of the mucosal flaps.

Augmentation pharyngoplasty (Hynes) *(Figure 8.4)*

This procedure also relies on the presence of muscle function, albeit more limited than for the Sommerlad rerepair and Furlow procedures. The goal of the procedure is to reduce the distance of travel for the soft palate to achieve closure of the velopharyngeal port. This is achieved by elevation of superiorly based flaps on the posterior pharyngeal wall, and suturing them together across the midline. This produces a bulge and, in addition, the closure of the flap donor sites produces a further reduction in the diameter of the port. This is more of a surgical insult and, although complications are uncommon, they can include flap loss and very noisy snoring. As with other pharyngoplasties, minor upper respiratory tract infections cause a blocked nose much more readily than normal

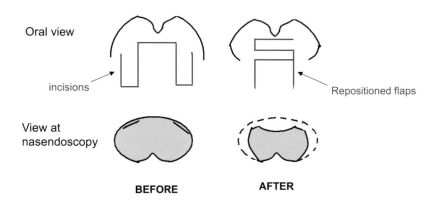

Figure 8.4: Hynes pharyngoplasty

Sphincter pharyngoplasty (Orticochea)

This procedure (see *Figure 8.5* produces the most predictable results as it is independent of palatal muscle function. The size of the velopharyngeal port is determined by the surgeon during the procedure and can, if necessary, be adjusted surgically at a later date. The procedure consists of elevating the posterior tonsillar fauces, overlapping them (Jackson's modification), and then insetting them into the posterior pharyngeal wall. The flaps contain muscle (palatopharyngeus) and the pharyngoplasty is claimed to be dynamic in nature, although this continues to be debated. Predictable in respect of benefit to speech, the price of permanent partial upper airways obstruction is equally predictable. Clearing the nose can be impossible

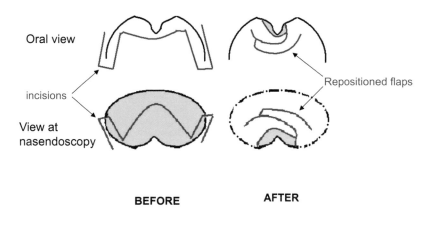

Figure 8.5: Orticochea pharyngoplasty

and any upper respiratory tract infection becomes a trial for both the patient and their relatives. There is also the risk of obstructive sleep apnoea, albeit that this is less than with flap pharyngoplasties.

Flap pharyngoplasties

These are static procedures which involve overlying flaps of mucosa from the posterior pharyngeal wall and the dorsal surface of the soft palate to partially obstruct the velopharyngeal port and enable closure to be achieved by action of the superior pharyngeal constrictor muscles. There are several port closure patterns apparent on nasendoscopy, and where the closure is from the sides towards the midline, there is logic to using this form of pharyngoplasty. The disadvantages are that they are totally passive/static flaps and tend to narrow with time, with loss of benefit. In addition, they are not anatomical and are the pharyngoplasty most frequently associated with obstructive sleep apnoea.

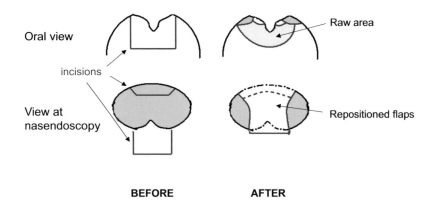

Figure 8.6: Flap pharyngoplasties

9
Pre and post operative nursing care

Vanessa Martin

Traditionally, babies with a cleft lip and palate had their lip repaired according to the rule of ten, i.e. when they weighed ten pounds, had reached the age of ten weeks and had haemoglobin of 10g. Now, with experienced paediatric anaesthetists, some surgeons are operating on babies' lips neonatally. Children with a cleft lip and palate are cared for in regional specialist cleft lip and palate units within a paediatric family-centred environment (Department of Health, 1991). An experienced team of paediatric nurses, with an appropriate backup team and facilities, is essential for the safety and well being of these infants. Kennedy (2001) recommended that health care professionals responsible for children should always hold a recognised qualification for their care. Facilities for parents are also required in hospital to ensure the least possible disruption to their family life.

Preoperative preparation

The employment of clinical nurse specialists to cleft teams provides the opportunity for families to be prepared for their hospital admission in their own home.

It is important that parents are prepared in advance for this stressful experience, which causes major disruption to their family life. Information leaflets dealing with all aspects of preparation, treatment, after care and potential problems should be provided (Action for Sick Children, 1996) and can be taken when the specialist visits. This may be an opportunity for the consent form to be explained, as recommended by the Department of Health. A visit to the ward before admission can be offered. Such a visit will help to orientate parents, familiarise them with facilities and equipment on the ward, with the route to the hospital, and identifying available parking.

The majority of children are admitted for surgery the day before their operation. Many units screen infants for group A beta-haemolytic streptococcal infection prior to admission, by sending nose and throat swabs for culture and sensitivity, as suggested by Armstrong *et al* (1993). GPs' surgeries may be asked to take these swabs and relay the result to the hospital, or they may be taken at pre-admission clinics. The virulent potential of this organism can break down wounds. In most units, the child will be started on oral antibiotics if swab results are positive. Rarely is there a need for surgery to be deferred.

On admission, photographic records of the cleft are obtained for the hospital notes. These show antero-posterior, inferior and lateral views and are needed to provide a baseline for follow up and audit purposes (CSAG, 1998).

An accurate weight of the infant for the calculation of anaesthetic and post operative drugs is recorded. Baseline observations of temperature, pulse, respiration and blood pressure are also documented, and a urine test obtained. Prior to a cleft palate repair, the child's assessment might include obtaining a full blood count and 'grouping and cross matching', although many anaesthetists now take blood from children when they are anaesthetised.

Arm splints have been widely used in the past to prevent interference with both the repair of the lip and palate, but have been shown to be of no apparent benefit (Jigjinni *et al*, 1993), particularly if the palate repair is undertaken at the earlier age of six months, rather than 14 to 18 months. In some units parents may choose whether or not to use arm splints, and occasionally surgeons request them.

Infants may have food and formula milk up to five hours and breast milk, water or weak juice up to two hours prior to surgery (Phillips *et al*, 1994). Many anaesthetists have a ruling of six hours and three hours, respectively, for these fluids. Children are bathed and dressed warmly in easily removable garments before surgery, and local anaesthetic cream is applied over suitable venous access sites unless contraindicated (Twycross *et al*, 1998).

The Department of Health recommends that parents are present during the induction of anaesthesia and during post operative recovery (Department of Health, 1996), although many hospitals still do not allow this. This is a traumatic time for parents and they need good preparation and support from the nursing staff.

Post operative care

Breathing

Regular assessment of the pulse and rate, and quality of the infant's respiration's following a primary repair of the cleft lip or palate should be made. It is very important to be aware that infants of less than six months of age are obligate nasal breathers (Advanced Life Support Group, 1997). An infant used to a large airway has to cope with a smaller one following the repair. Initial signs of an infant having airway difficulties are 'sucking in' of the lower lip on inspiration and sternal, intercostal, or sub costal recession. It is essential that these early signs of distress are acted upon promptly, as an infant's condition can deteriorate rapidly (Martin, 2001). Post operative airway obstruction can result from oedema, the presence of blood or exudate in the respiratory tract, or certain drugs. The anaesthetist should be alerted immediately, if there are concerns about the child's airway. Some children may benefit from nasal airways, particularly those that are operated on neonatally or following a complete bilateral cleft lip repair.

It is helpful to have the additional safeguard of an apnoea monitor and oxygen saturation monitor. It is usual for the saturation rate of an infant of two months to be between 97 and 100 per cent (Stebbens *et al*, 1991). The child should be laid on one side to allow blood and secretions to drain naturally from the mouth and nose. Suction should be used with caution, as the nose and palate are vulnerable to damage following surgery.

A safety measure that may be used in some units to guard the infant's airway is a tongue stitch (Millard, 1980). This consists of a silk suture, which is inserted into the posterior aspect of the tongue. Oral airways can irritate the palatal suture line, so a tongue stitch can be used to pull the tongue forward and open up the oral airway in an emergency. It is removed as soon as the child is fully alert. Many units have now ceased to use tongue stitches.

Nutrition

Following primary surgery, infants usually return from the theatre with a maintenance intravenous infusion of half strength Hartmann's solution, or 4% dextrose with 0.1% saline. In infants up to 10 kilograms, this will be infused at a 100mls per kilogram of body weight for 24 hours. Unless the lip is very bruised, a baby who has had a cleft lip repair will often take oral fluids soon after return from theatre. In most units, the infant is offered a normal feed either from the breast or their regular bottle as soon as they appear hungry. Infusions are discontinued once the infant's feeding regime is beginning to be restored.

Cleft palate surgery is more invasive, especially if both hard and soft palate clefts have been repaired, and infants are much more reluctant to drink. Rarely surgeons prefer infants to be fed with a spoon or cup following cleft palate surgery. The majority will be allowed to drink straight from their regular bottle or from the breast. Many units will allow a soft diet to begin from the morning following the operation. Infants are more likely to eat than they are to drink, as food appears much easier to swallow. Painkillers are given before meal times, as it is easier for infants to eat and drink if they are pain free. A nasogastric tube passed at the time of surgery can settle infants who are reluctant to drink. If fed by nasogastric tube the night after the operation, they appear to sleep better, to require a lower dose of opioids, and oral analgesia can be administered regularly and more easily (Kent, 2002).

Comfort

Following repair of a cleft lip, paracetamol usually settles infants comfortably, along with their normal bottle or breast feeds. An occasional dose of codeine phosphate or a non-steroidal anti-inflammatory drug (NSAID) may be needed if the lip is bruised.

Following repair of a cleft palate, especially if there is hard as well as soft palate involvement, infants can be very uncomfortable. A standard protocol has been developed, for drugs used in paediatric pain management, of opioids, codeine phosphate, NSAID and paracetamol (Twycross *et al*, 1998). If a combination of these is used, much greater pain relief effect will be produced than by using them individually. Similarly, a NSAID and paracetamol together produce a greater pain relief effect (Twycross *et al*, 1998).

According to Yaster and Maxwell (1993), doctors are still hesitant to prescribe opioids for children of less than one year old. They stress that, if opioids are needed, they should be given, but regular observation recordings and oxygen saturation monitoring is vital (Royal College of Paediatrics and Child Health, 1997; Yaster and Maxwell, 1993). Protocols of pain relief should be developed with the anaesthetists and audited regularly (CSAG, 1998). The opinion of parents on the adequacy of their child's pain relief should also be sought.

Safety

Lip care

As the presence of food and debris can cause infection, the care of the suture line following lip surgery is important. The wound should be cleaned with warmed normal saline. The formation of scabs should be discouraged, as the removal of scabs with the sutures will remove any new cells that have formed on the scar line (Miller, 1994). An application of antibiotic cream or soft paraffin helps to protect the area. Care of the lip suture line can be negotiated with parents and, if they agree, can be taught to them. In my experience, they will perform this diligently. It is important when cleaning to use a cotton bud in a gentle rolling action.

Sutures are removed on the fifth day, usually under sedation (Cuthbert, 1994), although occasionally in theatre, or in very young babies, when asleep after a feed. The removal of sutures is a skilled procedure, as great care is needed around the delicate columella and lip margin area. Some surgeons are now using Vicryl dissolvable sutures, which may take 3–4 weeks to dissolve completely.

Palate care

Regular fluids are necessary to keep the mouth moist and clean, attempting to create an environment that promotes healing (Miller, 1994). Sterile water should be given following milk, food and medicine. It is possible that bio yoghurt (with no lumps) given twice daily also aids the healing process by acting as a probotic. It is suggested that the use of probiotic bacteria promote a barrier mechanism in the body in babies with atopic dermatitis, food allergy and intestinal problems, acting as a treatment and prevention strategy (Isolauri *et al*, 2000; Majamaa and Isolauri, 1997; Saavedra *et al*, 1994). The perceived action of a probotic post surgery would be to coat the palatal mucosa with bacteria that are thought to be harmless, replacing any pathogens and preventing them colonising. More research is needed to prove the effectiveness of probiotics following cleft palate surgery. Analgesic suspensions and prophylactic antibiotics, if used, must be administered using sterile spoons and/or oral syringes to prevent hospital-acquired infections. The use of dummies is either discouraged from birth, or they are removed for a period of five weeks post-operatively (Cuthbert, 1994).

As the mouth is stretched open with a mouth gag during surgery, some infants develop sore areas at the lip angles. These can be soothed by regularly applying sterile soft paraffin, which stops the area cracking and attempts to create the ideal environment to accelerate wound healing (Miller, 1994). Soft paraffin can also be applied to dry lips.

Children should be discharged from hospital when they are eating and drinking and parents are confident about caring for them at home.

Children with syndromes

Children with a syndrome require a more detailed assessment pre-operatively, and may need to be seen prior to admission. Otherwise, they require similar pre and post operative care.

A proportion of children may have a tracheostomy. Their basic needs should, therefore, be negotiated even more thoroughly. It is important to acknowledge the experience parents have in the care of their child, and to define the role of the nurse and parent in hospital. Parents become very competent in caring for their child's tracheostomy at home, but need support while in a hospital environment. It is important to point out to them that the environment in a hospital is drier than that of the home. This means there is a greater potential for crusts to form inside the tracheostomy tube, which could be fatal (Serra *et al*, 1986). The administration of regular humidity is essential, and can be given through a 'Swedish Nose', a device that clips on to the end of the tube, and by the use of a humidifier. Suction should be given not only to remove secretions, but also to evaluate the patency of the tube. A spare tube, the same size as the child's tube, should always be ready with tapes attached in the event of an emergency. Staff responsible for a child with a tracheostomy should have been instructed in the procedure for changing the tube and have practised a tube change so that their first experience is not in an emergency situation (Martin, 2001)

Paediatricians should be aware of the admission of children with syndromes. This is especially important if the syndrome includes a heart defect, as the child's condition needs close monitoring post operatively.

Pierre Robin Sequence

Children with Pierre Robin Sequence may already have had surgery delayed to allow sufficient jaw development to ensure surgical access and preservation of the airway (Nottingham City Hospital, 1994). Parents of children with small mandibles have usually been warned that intubation may be difficult. Similarly, parents must be warned that, if their child had breathing difficulties and made inspiratory noises during the first weeks of his life, he may revert to making these noises immediately post operatively. This can last for about 12 hours while the child is accommodating to the new airway.

Children with Pierre Robin sequence need very careful observation post operatively. They may need overnight observation in intensive care or, if nursed in a paediatric ward, the on-call paediatric anaesthetist or paediatrician should be aware and available in case of an emergency.

Discharge advice

Cleft lip

Parents are encouraged to leave scabs that form on the child's lip following suture removal or around dissolvable sutures to drop off naturally. When the lip has healed totally, scar lines may be kept supple by massaging them twice daily with non-perfumed oil-based cream, for example, E45 Kamilosan or aqueous cream. This helps to break down the irregular pattern formation of collagen fibres in scar tissues (Bosworth, 1997; Gollup, 1997). Parents are asked to continue massaging the scar until it is white and mature. This may take up to a year. They are also warned that, on massaging, it is normal at first for pieces of stitch to come loose. This should not deter them from the massaging process. Parents whose child has had dissolvable sutures inserted may need to gently rub the suture line with gauze or a dry cotton bud after 10 days to begin to loosen the stitches.

Parents should be told to protect the scar from the sun by using a total sun block regularly, both in the morning and at lunchtime.

Cleft palate

On returning home, parents are asked, initially, to keep their child away from children or adults with coughs and colds and away from nursery schools and other crowded places. This is because children appear more vulnerable to infection in the immediate postoperative period.

Parents should be given advice on nourishing foods to give their child and when to return to a normal diet. The majority of units recommend a soft diet be continued for a month to six weeks following surgery (Cuthbert, 1994). Pulses are discouraged in the child's diet at first, as the skins can stick to the suture line. Fruit yoghurts with pips are also discouraged. Parents are asked to continue rinsing their child's mouth with water after food for at least two weeks and, if recommended, to continue using bio yoghurts to protect the wound.

In units using arm splints, children may have to continue wearing them at home for a few weeks especially when they are not being supervised and at night (Berkowitz, 1994).

Care of the child admitted for alveolar bone grafting

Alveolar bone graft surgery is performed by the maxillofacial surgeon. The time is dictated by the eruption of the canine tooth in children with clefts that involve the primary palate. Cancellous bone is harvested, usually from the anterior iliac crest, and packed into the area of the alveolar defect following repair of the floor of the nose and of any palatal fistula. A mucoperiosteal flap is used to secure the bone grafted site. Within three months of successful surgery, grafts appear to be indistinguishable radiologically and behave clinically as normal alveolar bone (Mars, 2001).

Alveolar bone graft surgery usually takes place at the age of 9 to 11 years. Both the patient and parents will be anxious about this hospital admission, and will need careful preparation. A visit to the ward, and leaflets or a booklet dealing with all aspects of preparation, treatment, and aftercare should be given prior to admission. Contact with a family who have already experienced this operation is often helpful.

Preoperative preparation

This will vary according to the surgeon and may include the sending of nose swabs for culture and sensitivity, and bloods for a full blood count. Photographs are taken as a baseline for follow up, and will include the upper dental arch and nose. The latter is helpful for assessing whether the bone graft has improved the contour of the alar base. A chlorhexidine gluconate (Corsodyl®) mouth wash may also be given preoperatively.

Post operative care

The patient may return to the ward with dressing plates and occasionally arch wires in position (see *Chapter 11*). There will usually be a Mefix® dressing to the hip wound. Intravenous opiates may be given as post operative analgesia, but as the hip is usually the most painful, topical anaesthetic in the form of bupivicaine (Marcain®) into the iliac crest may be used as an alternative. This is given either as a continuous, or bolus infusion via an intravenous cannular inserted through the skin posterior to the wound site (Dunstan and Korezak, 1996). Antibiotics may be given intravenously post operatively. Regimes for drinking and eating may vary, as some surgeons are concerned that fluid and diet given too early may lead to a greater risk of infection in the grafted site. Patients should be on a normal diet by the second post operative day, and should be ready for discharge home.

It is essential that nurses are confident about teaching oral hygiene to the patient before discharge, and that the importance of this is stressed. Gentle brushing of teeth and gums with a soft tooth brush, even around the grafted area, should be done regularly, especially after meals. Extra special attention to brushing is required if an arch wire is present. Plenty of fluids should be encouraged, and chlorhexidine gluconate mouth washes given three times a day. Antibiotics are usually continued orally at home for a further five days.

Patients are encouraged to be up and walking on the first post operative day, and to mobilise regularly to aid the early return to normal function, if callous bone has been harvested from the iliac crest. The continuous suture is removed from the hip wound as an outpatient, and patients are advised to return to school when they are feeling fit. They are advised to refrain from active sports for a week or two after returning.

Care of the young adult requiring orthognathic surgery

A small proportion of young adults may require orthognathic surgery. This is due to the under-development of the maxilla. Surgery often involves a Le Fort 1 maxillary osteotomy, when the mandible is separated at Le Fort 1 level and moved forward to aid normal occlusion of the teeth. It is fixed in its new position using titanium plates and screws. Occasionally, patients may return from theatre with arch wires or elastics to stabilise the new jaw position. In these cases, a high dependency bed may be needed for the first postoperative night.

Preoperative care

Preoperative photographs are taken as a baseline for follow up and audit, and bloods are taken for a full blood count. Patients are prepared for post operative swelling and nausea and a possible nasal airway. They are seen by a dietician who will advise on post operative nutrition and arrange for a fluid diet. The patient will also be instructed on mouth care and dental hygiene.

Post operative care

Breathing

It is important to ensure that oxygen and suction are available at the bedside post operatively and that if the jaws are wired, wire cutters are available in case of an emergency.

The patient should be nursed upright to assist in reducing oral swelling and, if a nasal airway is present, this should be suctioned 1–2 hourly to ensure its patency.

Comfort

Patients often return from theatre with opiates in the form of patient controlled analgesia (PCA).

Swelling

Patients are prescribed intravenous dexamethasone to help reduce facial swelling. Regular applications of hydrocortisone ointment may have been applied to lips throughout surgery to reduce trauma, and may be prescribed post operatively.

Nausea and vomiting

Anti-emetics are usually prescribed intravenously. Patients should be instructed that if they vomit, they should lean forward over a vomit bowl and try to blow out through their mouth. Suction should be used to the nasal and oral cavities.

Mouth care

Antibiotics are usually prescribed intravenously for 48 hours to reduce the risk of infection. Chlorhexidine gluconate mouth washes are prescribed 2 to 4 hourly. The importance of brushing teeth with a soft toothbrush, as soon as possible following surgery, should be stressed to patients. Tooth brushing and the drinking of plenty of clear fluids should be encouraged, following milk and diet, once these are started.

Patients may need the assistance of a dental hygienist, if one is available, especially if their teeth are wired.

If hydrocortisone ointment is not prescribed for the lips, then regular Vaseline® should be applied to prevent drying.

Nutrition

Fluids are given to the patient as they are tolerated, and a fluid diet will gradually progress to a soft diet as the pain and swelling reduce.

The dietician should be involved in ensuring a nourishing diet that is tolerated by the patient. If the patient's jaw is wired, it is important to discourage him/her from poking food like chips through the gaps as these cannot be retrieved if there should be a problem.

On discharge:

- Patients are warned of the risk of vomiting should they drink alcohol, and advised not to smoke

- X-rays are performed to check the new jaw positions

- Photographs are taken once the swelling has subsided

- Arch wires may remain for between one and three weeks

- Plates and screws will not be removed unless they cause a problem.

10
Speech and language difficulties associated with cleft palate

Lorraine Britton

Introduction

It has been recognised that children with cleft palate are at high risk of both speech disorders and language delay (Russell and Harding, 2001). Historically, up to 40% of children in the UK, who had a cleft, developed communication difficulties requiring speech and language therapy (Enderby, 1986). Consequently, the speech and language therapist (SLT) plays a key role in any cleft team.

Role of the speech and language therapist

The role of the SLT in the cleft team includes:
- Monitoring speech and language development
- Identifying cleft related speech difficulties and investigating whether the difficulties are due to the anatomy of the oral cavity (structural), or the way the child has learned to talk (functional), or both
- Providing therapy
- Liaising closely with other members of the team to ensure appropriate care
- Auditing speech outcomes.

Speech

The term 'speech' is used by SLTs to describe the sounds, articulation patterns, resonance and voice used in speaking

(Morley, 1970). A child's speech pattern can be delayed or disordered, and this may or may not affect the meanings the child wishes to convey. For example, a child who says 't' instead of 's' will not be able to convey the difference between the words 'sew' and 'toe', whereas a lisped 's' is unlikely to interfere with meaning.

Voice is produced in the larynx (voice box) by the vibration of exhaled air through the vocal folds. This is subsequently modified through resonance of the air in the pharyngeal, nasal, and oral cavities. The vowels of speech are particularly influenced by voice and resonance.

In speech articulation, the lips, tongue, vocal folds, and soft palate all work together to modify the exhaled air to produce each of the consonants and vowels used in any given language. These articulators all move extremely quickly to create the patterns of sounds used in words to convey meaning and, therefore, enable effective communication. To help you think about this , consider the word:

◆ **COSMOPOLITAN**

Think about what your lips, tongue, vocal folds, and soft palate are doing for each of the consonant sounds.

In English, there are 24 consonant sounds, which create differences in meaning (phonemes). Of these, only three are nasal consonants. The rest are oral consonants, which are normally produced with the soft palate raised to close off the velopharyngeal port. This closure is of particular importance for the consonants requiring a build up of oral pressure shown below.

	Nasal (soft palate lowered)	Oral (soft palate raised)	
		Voiceless	Voiced
Lips closed	m	p	b
Lips and teeth		f	v
Tongue at front	n	t	d
		s/sh	z
Tongue at back	ng	k	g

Articulation is an acquired motor skill, developing gradually in childhood and dependent on the anatomy and physiology of the articulatory apparatus, accurate neurological control, and good sensory feedback.

Cleft type speech

Children born with a cleft palate are at high risk of developing a range of disordered patterns of speech, as a result of their disturbed anatomy and associated medical problems. For example, when:

- The soft palate does not close off the velopharyngeal port effectively

- There is a fistula or unrepaired cleft

- There are orthodontic or occlusal problems

- There is chronic or fluctuating hearing loss.

The nature of cleft-type speech characteristics and their structural influences are well described in the literature (Grunwell and Sell, 2001; Harding and Grunwell, 1996).

Children with cleft are also prone to the same range of developmental speech difficulties exhibited by other children. These may be intertwined with cleft type speech characteristics. It is the role of the SLT to tease this out.

Assessing cleft-type speech

When assessing the speech of a person with a history of cleft palate, the SLT will consider three key factors:

1. **Resonance**: How is the balance of air resonating in the oral/nasal cavities?

2. **Articulation**: Are the speech sounds produced correctly?

3. **Intelligibility**: Can we understand him?

Alongside these key factors, the therapist will also assess a patient's language, comprehension, voice, and overall communication skills in relation to their developmental level.

The main form of speech assessment is skilled and detailed perceptual assessment. In the UK, the most common tool used for this is the GOS.SP.ASS. '98 (Sell *et al*, 1999). Alongside this, there are now more objective measurement tools, including the nasometer and electropalatograph.

The **resonance** refers to the balance of air resonating in the oral and nasal cavities. A person is described as being 'hypernasal' if there is too much air resonating in the nasal cavity and 'hyponasal' if there is too little air.

Hypernasality is often associated with a soft palate which is unable to close off the velopharyngeal port effectively, leading to excessive air in the nasal cavity and heard, particularly on vowels and voiced consonants. This is known as velopharyngeal dysfunction. It is a common complication following cleft palate, but is also seen in the non cleft population. Associated symptoms often include: nasal regurgitation of food, difficulties with sucking or blowing, audible nasal emission, nasal turbulence, and voice problems. Speech often sounds better with nose holding.

Hyponasality is often the result of a nasal blockage. This may be temporary, e.g. due to a cold, or more long term, e.g. due to enlarged adenoids, deviated septum, or allergy. It is heard particularly on nasal consonants. This is less commonly associated with cleft palate. Associated symptoms may include snoring and mouth breathing. Speech is not usually improved with nose holding.

Problems with **resonance** are often structural and cannot usually be corrected by speech and language therapy alone.

In considering **articulation**, there are a number of common cleft-type speech characteristics. The CAPS audit tool (Harding *et al*, 1997) lists the following ten most common:

Characteristic	'Fools Guide'
Lateralisation	slushy 's, z'
Palatalisation	slushy 's, z, t, d'
Backing to velar	t→k, d–g, e.g. 'table→cable', 'daddy→gaggy'
Backing to uvular	a bit further back than velar
Pharyngeal	throaty sounds
Glottal	produced by the vocal folds—lazy 't'
Weak nasalised consonants	
Nasal realisations	b→m, e.g. 'ball→mall'; d→n, e.g. 'daddy→nanny'
Absent pressure consonants	mainly vowels heard, e.g. 'daddy' 'a→ee'
Active nasal fricative	air forced down nose on specific sounds—often 's'

There are thought to be some common associations between speech patterns and structural anomalies (Russell and Harding, 2001: 196):

◆ Lateralisation/palatalisation are commonly associated with dental and occlusal anomalies

◆ Backing is commonly associated with fistulae

◆ Nasal realisations are commonly associated with velopharyngeal dysfunction

◆ Active nasal fricatives are commonly associated with conductive hearing loss.

Problems with articulation will often require speech and language therapy, either with or without surgery to correct them.

Intelligibility is a rather subjective measure of how easily we can understand a child. It is influenced by a range of variables relating to the speaker, listener and environment and, therefore, has to be interpreted cautiously.

Management of speech problems

Following detailed speech assessment, recommendations will be made concerning further management. If the speech pattern is indicative of a structural problem, such as velopharyngeal dysfunction, the child will be referred for objective assessment of palate function using lateral videofluoroscopy and/or nasendoscopy with a view to further surgery as appropriate.

If the problem is functional, speech and language therapy will be offered alongside, or instead of, surgical intervention. Therapy may work on any aspect of communication, including: language development, social skills, comprehension, attention and listening, parent-child interaction, as well as the more obvious speech sound production.

Therapy often takes some time and requires an educational/social model of care, rather than a medical model. It is, therefore, likely to be provided at a local level wherever possible, sometimes working directly with the child or through the school or parents.

Where a child needs help with articulation, therapy is often based on the following principles:

- Work from the sounds the child finds easiest

- Focus on ensuring correct place of articulation

- Listening and looking before production

- Minimise pressure to produce wherever possible.

General advice relating to early speech development (up to 2.5 years)

Some SLT experts advocate early intervention to try to prevent the development of speech and language problems (Golding-Kushner, 2001; Russell and Harding, 2001). Furthermore, it is known that parents who are anxious about their child's speech and language development are likely to spontaneously adapt the way they talk to their child. The following strategies may be suggested to try to ensure that any adaptations parents make are constructive:

- Encourage babble play and making noises (i.e. animal noises) to help the baby discover what his new mouth can do after surgery

- Have babble 'conversations'. Copy the sounds the baby makes and make new sounds for him to watch and maybe try (Ward, 2000)

- Make noises onto babies' bodies to help them to see, hear and feel the sounds, e.g. blow gently into their hair with a 'fffff' or blow raspberries on their tummy. If they like it, they may attempt the sound to ask for more

- Easy first sounds are the nasals 'm/n' and, therefore, words like 'mummy' and 'no'

- Early sounds we hope to hear by 18 months are 'b/d/g' and early words like 'bye, boo, daddy' and 'gone'. These can be encouraged by frequent repetition and modelling

- Speak normally and avoid over-exaggerating the sounds, or shouting

- Discourage glottal stops (often mistaken for b/d/g), and unusual nasal sounds by ignoring

At first, the child's words will not be clear. Do not worry. Gently model back the words they are trying to say, but do not ask them to correct their production.

If the child's speech continues to be difficult to understand, ensure (s)he sees a speech and language therapist for more personally tailored advice.

Language

Speech and language therapists define a child's language skills as the ability to learn, understand and use words and to combine these using the correct grammatical rules to formulate sentences and conversations. Children's language skills develop alongside their speech. Children can have difficulties either with understanding or using language. Again these difficulties may be delayed or disordered.

Children with cleft are known to be at high risk of language delay (Russell and Harding, 2001: 193). This has been related to a range of factors, including associated conductive hearing problems, lower parental expectations and disrupted parent-child interaction patterns. Typically, children will say their first words at around 12–18 months of age and begin combining words at around 2 years. These milestones may be later for children with clefts.

General advice relating to early language development (up to 2.5 years)

Given that young children with cleft are at risk of language delay, the following strategies, which have been reported in the literature to help language development, may be useful (Golding-Kushner, 2001; Ward, 2000; Manolson, 1992):

- Follow the baby's lead in play
- Comment on what the baby is doing throughout daily routines
- Speak to the baby in single words at first then short simple sentences
- Add meaning to the baby's vocalisations
- Offer choices 'juice' or 'milk'
- Reduce background noise, e.g. TV, where possible
- Encourage make-believe play from 18 months onwards, e.g. tea parties
- Encourage parents to enjoy singing and nursery rhymes with their baby
- Encourage understanding as well as speech, e.g. ask the child to point out things in a book, or wash named body parts
- Discourage parents from using lots of questions
- Watch favourite videos together and listen for certain words or songs
- Look at picture books together.

If the language problems persist, ensure (s)he sees a speech and language therapist for more personally tailored advice.

Summary

This chapter provides a brief overview of the range of speech and language difficulties commonly associated with cleft lip and palate. It has also outlined the role of the SLT with children with cleft, and provided information on early advice that might be offered. For a more detailed description, the reader is referred to the relevant chapters in Watson *et al* (2001).

11
Dental health care and orthodontics

Dental health

Patricia Bannister

Although some young people have had no experience of tooth decay, recent surveys show that this continues to remain a serious problem for many children and adults. Such problems are easily preventable and, as with other members of the cleft team, a nurse involved in the care of a child and his/her family has a responsibility to assist in the prevention of dental disease.

Within the first few weeks following the birth of a cleft child, parents will inevitably ask questions as to their child's dental development and the need for treatment in the future. Likely questions may revolve around teething, the appearance of the teeth around the cleft site, their position in the gums and how this arrangement is likely to affect the appearance of the growing child. From this early stage, it is important that parents understand their role in the value of good dental health, and begin to consider how, as parents, they will approach this potential problem. This will often involve the nuclear and extended family, particularly if older siblings already have entrenched eating patterns. Safeguarding oral health in infancy and childhood is likely to lead to good oral health in adulthood (Powell, 1998). National targets in a recent NHS plan (Department of Health, 2000) have suggested that a national target of no more than one decayed, missing or filled tooth for all 5-year-olds should be achieved by 2003.

Specific dental problems related to cleft lip and palate

- Absent or supernumary teeth

- Misshapen teeth

- Hypo plastic enamel; seen in 24% of teeth around the cleft site (Chapple *et al*, 2001)

- Malposition of teeth

- Malocclusion and misalignment of teeth

- During the use of orthodontic appliances.

Educating parents

A recent published survey showed that a simple community oral health programme, aimed at parents with young children, can reduce dental decay substantially (Kowash, 2000). Such programmes should not be the sole responsibility of the dental profession and can be effectively undertaken by health visitors/nurses, general practitioners, or any member of the cleft team. It appears important that verbal instruction takes into consideration the knowledge base of the parents and existing family behaviour. This may be supplemented by written information and an agreed plan of care, which considers realistic goals for any given family. The details of such a plan can be documented in the section on dental health in the parent-held records. Achievable plans may include: absence of dietary sugar, control of sugar attacks, daily tooth brushing, registration and regular assessment by a dental practitioner, and the use of a variety of fluoride treatments. Any preventive management must revolve around regular dental checkups, effective and frequent tooth brushing, and dietary advice.

Tooth brushing

The need to educate families with young children on the importance of tooth brushing is becoming increasingly recognised. Children do not have the manual dexterity to brush their own teeth properly until they are 6–7 years of age. However, it is important too that children are encouraged to help in the brushing of their teeth. Parents may be nervous about brushing teeth in the region of the cleft, especially following primary surgery, alveolar bone grafting, and orthognathic surgery. They need to be shown how to brush the teeth and gums properly, and given the opportunity to practice the technique in the home, hospital, and dental surgery (Rifkin *et al*, 2000). Particular periods when parents may need help are:

- Eruption of first tooth
- Post operatively following primary surgery
- As the child takes on the task of cleaning his/her own teeth
- Pre and post alveolar bone grafting
- During orthodontic treatment
- Following orthognathic surgery.

Tooth brushes vary in size and shape and Rifkin *et al* (2000) suggests, that a small head is ideal where there is a lack of sulcus depth in the upper lip, and the additional use of an interspace brush where there is overlap, overcrowding, and/or retroclined incisors, often observed where there is a bilateral cleft lip and palate. She also describes in detail the ideal position for a parent to hold a child when assisting in tooth brushing. The use of fluoride toothpaste is now recommended for all children, and Roch (1994) recommends toothpaste of no more than 600ppm fluoride for children under the age of six years. Children at high risk of dental decay can be advised to use a standard adult toothpaste containing a 1000ppm fluoride. The use of fluoride supplements and other dental treatments will largely depend on detailed discussions with the parents and the fluoride content of the local water supply. Advice about the latter can be obtained from the local health authority or dental practitioner.

Dietary advice

One of the main contributories to severe tooth decay in young children is the inappropriate use of feeding bottles, the learned habit of grazing, eating and drinking small amounts frequently throughout the day, and the free availability of sugary foods and drinks. As the young baby moves towards the age of weaning, bottles of sweet drinks are often available to the child at all times of the day and are sometimes used as a pacifier. The enamel on the tooth is exposed to sugar for long periods of time and does not have sufficient time to recover. Additionally, the normal protective flow of saliva virtually ceases during sleep, making teeth more susceptible to decay during these times (Department of Health, 2000).

A similar affect on tooth enamel may be seen as the infant moves away from routine four hourly meal times and slots into family eating patterns. If there are no regular family meal times, children learn to graze, eating or drinking at frequent intervals throughout the day. Snack foods and drinks are often those with a high sugar content. Such habits learned in childhood are often continued into the teenage years.

Good dietary management

- Use of cool boiled water if require between milk feeds
- Limited use of well diluted juice
- Confine juice and sweet foods to mealtimes in older toddlers and children and use water for thirst between meals
- Encourage three to four meals a day
- Confine sugar free snacks to twice daily
- Avoid the use of a dummy dipped in a sugary substance
- Encourage the discussion of the importance of good dental health with other members of the family and carers.

The older child

As a child grows older, he or she must learn to accept responsibility for his/her own dental health. Children will need help in understanding how to achieve this, as difficulties in tooth brushing and dietary planning become evident. Anxieties around eruption of the second dentition, bleeding from the gingivai in the region of the cleft should be identified. Oral health related to bone grafting is important in preventing the loss of the implanted bone, especially during the first 10 to 14 days after surgery (see *Chapter 10*).

Nurse's role

- Identify responsibility of the parent
- Identify parental knowledge base and family oral health
- Establish team responsibility in approach
- Pace and target advice from infancy to adulthood
- Reinforce/explain advice following clinic appointments
- Consider damage limitation
- Understand family functioning
- Ensure registration with local dental services.

Messages about oral health need to be kept simple, and family and age appropriate. Parents and children are the main custodians of healthy dentition and their responsibility needs to be clearly stated. Support and advice is the responsibility of every health professional, with the dental practitioner and oral hygienist having a key role in this aspect of care.

Orthodontics in cleft lip and palate

Gunvor Semb and Bill Shaw

O rthodontics is the branch of dentistry that deals with facial growth, development of the dentition and the occlusion, diagnosis, interception and treatment of occlusal anomalies.

Provided that space is available, the orthodontist may move a tooth in any direction, within cancellous bone and over a considerable distance. However, the possibility to influence facial growth is limited (Profitt, 1993). Orthodontic treatment is often a lengthy procedure (1 to 4 years) and is not without risks. Thus the benefits and risks must be discussed with the patient and the parents before starting the treatment (Shaw, 1993).

The orthodontic specialist responsible for the care of children with cleft lip and palate (CLP) must have an appreciation of the overall burden of care that children with clefts endure. The nature of dental development and impairment of facial growth in patients with repaired clefts is such that there may be temptations to intervene at almost any point between birth and the end of the teens. Consequently, clear choices must be made and orthodontic treatment that does not significantly contribute to the end result should be eliminated from the programme of care. The overall aim of treatment is to provide a dentition that functions well and is capable of lifetime maintenance by routine oral hygiene and dental care.

As a member of the multidisciplinary team, it is important to monitor the patient's general well-being, particularly during the years of greater involvement, 7–16 years.

Facial growth

Problems in facial growth are most commonly found in children with complete clefts of the lip and palate and are characterised by maxillary growth impairment in all three dimensions (Dahl, 1970; Enemark *et al*, 1990; Ross and Johnston, 1972; Semb and Shaw, 1996). The scar tissue formed, following traumatic primary surgery, can seriously affect the growth of the maxilla, with the antero-posterior growth of the maxilla causing the biggest problem. Patients, especially those born with complete cleft lip and palate may, in their teens, develop a straight or concave facial profile instead of the normal convex shape (see *Figure 11.1*). If the maxilla is seriously affected, the treatment the orthodontist can do is very limited, and jaw surgery is necessary if the patient wants improved occlusion and facial appearance. Orthodontists in the cleft team develop a close working

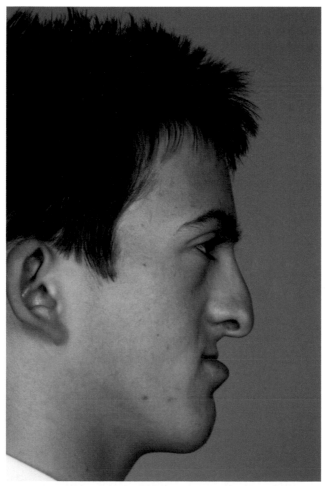

Figure 11.1: Profile view of a patient born with complete unilateral cleft lip and palate. Maxillary growth has been severely impaired and has left him with a concave facial profile.

relationship with surgeons in agreeing the surgery with the least traumatic long-term outcome

Dental development

Disturbances in dental development when a cleft of the alveolus is present produce variations in number, morphology, enamel formation, and eruption of teeth in the cleft area, with the lateral incisor (the small side-tooth in the frontal region) being most affected (BØhn, 1963; Ranta, 1986).

Lateral incisor

In the primary dentition, the lateral incisor is congenitally missing in 12–14% of cases, while in the permanent dentition, the lateral incisor is missing in about 45% of cases. When present, the lateral incisors may be found on either side of the alveolar cleft or, in case of supernumerary incisors, on both sides. In most cases, it is malformed.

Central incisor

The permanent central incisor (the large front tooth) on the cleft side is, on average, 10% narrower than the other central incisor, and its shape is often abnormal. In patients with bilateral CLP, they are frequently malformed and have a short root length.

Canine

The morphology of the canine does not appear to be affected by the occurrence of a cleft.

Occlusal development

It is quite common for patients with clefts to have crossbites, which means that the upper teeth bite on the inside of the lower teeth. Patients with clefts often have crossbite, both in the front (anterior crossbite) and in the lateral segments (lateral crossbite) (see Figure 11.2). This is mainly due to the scar tissue produced at primary surgery that pull erupting upper teeth palatally, reducing the maxillary dental arch.

In the primary dentition in children with complete unilateral cleft lip and palate (UCLP), crossbite of one or more teeth

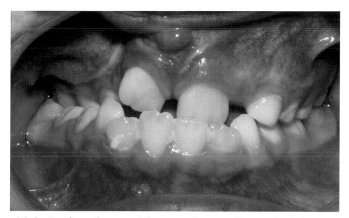

Figure 11.2: Patient born with complete unilateral cleft lip and palate. View of the occlusion show both anterior and unilateral crossbites

on the cleft side is the most common deviation from normal dental arch form. In some instances, anterior crossbite may also be found.

In children with complete bilateral cleft lip and palate (BCLP), the premaxilla is usually quite prominent during the primary dentition stage, but recedes over time. Since mandibular growth will later catch up with the premaxilla, it is important to resist the temptation to set back the premaxilla surgically. Bilateral crossbites are quite common.

The transition from deciduous to the mixed dentition is characterised by a worsening of the anterior occlusion, due to the palatal path of eruption and the rotation of the incisors adjacent to the cleft (Bergland and Sidhu, 1974).

As further development of the permanent dentition takes place, scar tissue in the palate may cause the permanent canines and premolars to erupt in a palatal direction. As a consequence of the shorter dental arches, crowding commonly develops in the posterior dentition when all teeth are present. In patients with unilateral CLP, the maxillary dental midline tends to be displaced to the cleft side, exaggerating the asymmetry of the face (Semb and Shaw, 2001).

Orthodontic treatment of complete cleft lip and palate

Principles

Formerly, the aims of the orthodontic treatment for children with complete clefts were limited to tooth alignment and arch expansion, followed by permanent artificial retention in the form of fixed bridgework or other prostheses. This was often linked with artificial restoration of the lateral incisor space, as the alveolar bony defect made orthodontic space closure impossible. This approach, however, had several disadvantages for, in addition to the general undesirability of artificial teeth for long-term aesthetics and dental health, lack of investing bone often precluded the correction of the anterior irregularities. Lack of supporting bone could also lead to so much loss of attachment of teeth adjacent to the cleft that they were lost after some years, and in patients with bilateral clefts, the mobility of the premaxilla made the retention of bridgework difficult (Semb and Shaw, 2001).

With the advent of a successful alveolar bone grafting technique in the early 1970s, the aims of treatment have been revised so that the alveolar bony defect is restored before the time of canine eruption (in the majority of cases). Subsequent orthodontic treatment can then achieve alignment, and a complete dental arch without false teeth can be obtained in the majority of cases (Bergland *et al*, 1986; Boyne and Sands, 1976; Enemark *et al*, 1987; Mars, 2001). The following simplified approach to treatment has provided satisfactory results. Because of the doubtful benefits of presurgical orthopaedics, deciduous dentition treatment and attempted skeletal protraction, and the unnecessary burden of care they impose, these interventions will not be recommended. We do not recommend the use of removable appliances.

Orthodontics prior to bone grafting

Incisor alignment

By age 7–8 years, an increased awareness of dental appearance and the motivation for orthodontic treatment often becomes evident. Incisor alignment can be provided at this stage, if requested for aesthetic reasons. Correction of inverted and rotated incisors will take between 3–6 months. A small bonded retainer is placed on the palatal aspects of the corrected incisors and is kept in place until the start of permanent dentition treatment (Semb and Shaw, 2001).

Orthodontic movement of maxillary anterior teeth at this time must, however, be done with great caution because of the closeness of the roots to the bony defect, and in some patients treatment is better postponed until after the alveolar process has been completely restored by bone.

Transverse expansion

If possible, transverse expansion can be combined with the correction of incisor irregularities, but expansion prior to bone grafting should not be regarded as essential for all crossbites. Only cases with significant segmental displacement require pre-bone graft expansion to facilitate placement of the graft. Most often, a removable quadhelix is used for segment repositioning, as selective expansion anteriorly is required (see *Figures 11.3.a and 3.b*). Segment repositioning will take approximately 4–8 months (Semb and Shaw, 2001).

Expansion may produce a slight widening of the nasal cavity in the antero-inferior region, but there is no evidence that this is permanently maintained. It is, therefore, likely that a significant improvement in nasal airflow occurs in only a small number of patients (Ross and Johnston, 1972). However, expansion of a severely constricted maxilla in the mixed dentition period may provide greater space for the tongue and improve speech articulation and masticatory function.

In patients with complete BCLP, the premaxilla may be mobile, and stabilisation of the premaxilla immediately before grafting has been found to improve the success of bone grafting. A heavy rectangular archwire is used for this and kept in place for three months after surgery (Semb and Shaw, 2001).

Timing of bone grafting

The optimum time of bone grafting is decided individually. In patients with a well formed lateral incisor, bone grafting

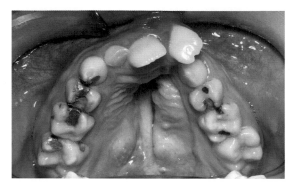

a) Before any orthodontic treatment

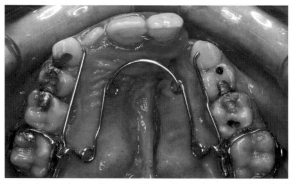

b) After the incisors have been aligned and a small twistflex retainer has been bonded on the palatal aspect of the incisors. The displacement of the lateral segment has been corrected by a removable quad helix. Total treatment time: 6 months

Figure 11.3: The maxillary arch of a patient born with complete unilateral cleft lip and palate

is usually done quite early, around 7–8 years. Since the majority of patients have a missing, displaced, or deformed lateral incisor, bone grafting may be postponed until 10–11 years. This allows the canine's root-development to progress more and may make canine eruption easier. However, grafting should still be performed prior to canine eruption. Female secondary dentition may erupt earlier than that of the male (Bergland *et al*, 1986; Mars, 2001).

Post surgical stabilisation

The quad helix and/or stabilising archwire used in BCLP may be removed during the bone grafting procedure for improved surgical access, but these appliances should be replaced before the patient leaves the operating theatre, and left in place for three months. When a substantial outward movement of the lateral segment(s) has been necessary, clinical experience suggests that bone grafting alone cannot be relied upon to maintain the expansion. In these circumstances, stabilisation in the form of a simple palatal arch would be advisable until the permanent dentition has erupted (Semb and Shaw, 2001).

Post-bone graft observation

Resting the patient from appliance therapy is highly desirable at this stage. Occasional observation is generally all that is necessary in the years between bone grafting and eventual eruption of the permanent dentition at around 12–13 years of age. The status of unerupted teeth, especially the cleft side canine, does, however, need careful monitoring.

Permanent dentition orthodontics

A number of special considerations make orthodontic treatment of children with complete clefts distinctive from general orthodontics.

● Deteriorating in the relationship between the upper and lower jaw

◆ Early determination of the eventual need for jaw surgery because of impaired maxillary growth is the most difficult and important decision for the orthodontist. Where the likelihood of jaw surgery is high, simple alignment of the upper arch may be all that is required until the end of the teens when a period of orthodontic treatment before the jaw surgery is necessary

- Absent lateral incisors
    - When maxillary lateral incisors are absent, two options present—orthodontic space closure, or space preservation for a replacement of various kinds.

In the author's opinion, orthodontic space closure so that the canine occupies the lateral incisor's position is generally the first choice, since the natural dentition has the best prognosis for long-term health. It is easy to reshape the crown of the canine to make it look more like a front tooth. Successful space closure relieves the patient of the burden of having false teeth and the associated lifetime maintenance (see *Figures 11.4.a; 4.b; 4.c; 5.a; 5.b*).

However, in patients with severely impaired maxillary growth and multiple missing teeth, orthodontic space closure may not be feasible.

Surgical transplantation of teeth can now be regarded as a treatment with high reliability in suitable cases. Premolars are suitable candidates for transplantation. Periodontal and pulp healing is best achieved, if transplantation is carried out when root development is half to three-quarters complete (Andreasen, 1992).

Unfortunately, the maxillary lateral incisor region may be an unsuitable site for single tooth implant. Continued growth precludes the placement of an implant until the end of growth, during which time the alveolar process reduces in height and volume, often requiring a further bone graft. For these reasons, implants are especially unsuited to the lateral incisor region, and their use in this setting should await further long-term follow-up studies (Semb and Shaw, 2001).

- Retention
    - The relapse tendency in patients with clefts is great compared to non-clefts, and is directly related to scar tissue from primary surgery. Thus, a tight upper lip and scars in the palate may encourage the migration of teeth into crossbite (Ross and Johnston, 1972). However, apart from the use of a bonded retainer extending to at least one tooth either side of the cleft, we considered lifetime use of retainers undesirable.

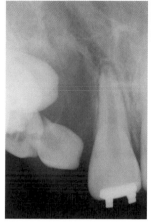

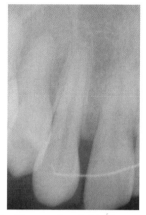

b) Radiograph of the former cleft area 12 years after bone grafting and 6 years after orthodontic completion

a) Radiograph of the alveolar bony defect before bone grafting

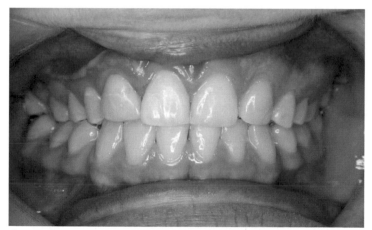

c) Frontal view of the occlusion 6 years after orthodontic completion

Figure 11.4: Patient born with complete unilateral cleft lip and palate (frontal view of teeth before any orthodontic treatment is show in Figure 11.2)

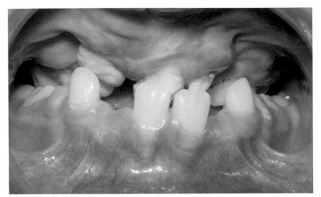

**a) Frontal view of the occlusion before any orthodontic
treatment**

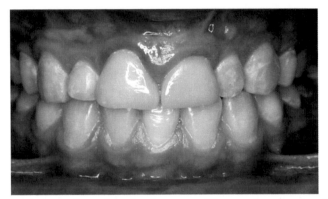

**b) Frontal view after alveolar bone grafting and orthodontic
treatment. Porcelain veneers have been placed on the central
incisors that were hypoplastic and deformed, and the lateral
incisors have had composite build-up for the same reason. One
incisor in the lower jaw has been extracted**

**Figure 11.5: Patient born with complete bilateral cleft lip and
palate**

- Unfavourable conditions for maxillary osteotomy

  - Orthognathic surgery in patients with repaired clefts
    requires especially careful planning between orthodon-
    tist, surgeon, and speech therapist. Maxillary
    osteotomy is technically more challenging because of

the underlying maxillary deformity, the presence of scarring, and the high relapse tendency—regardless of the means of fixation; the velopharyngeal mechanism may be adversely affected by maxillary advancement (Lello, 2001).

Other cleft types

Cleft lip and alveolus (CLA)

Since patients with CLA have normal maxillary growth, they can be treated according to orthodontic principles for non-clefts. But even though the alveolar arch at birth seems little affected by the cleft, in most instances irregularities of the number, size, shape, and form of the lateral incisor on the cleft side will be found.

Some patients with CLA have an alveolar bony defect large enough to restrict orthodontic closure of the space in the cleft region and, in these cases, alveolar bone grafting may be required.

Cleft palate only (CPO)

In patients with CPO, both maxilla and the mandible are smaller and more retrusive than in non-clefts. However, in most instances, the degree of retrusion is similar in both jaws and, therefore, the relationship between the jaws is usually satisfactory. Patients with CPO also have a higher frequency of missing teeth than their non-cleft counterparts. The dental arches are slightly narrower and shorter and dental crowding is a common feature. However, conventional orthodontics, often including extraction of teeth in both jaws, usually achieves an acceptable occlusion (Semb and Shaw, 2001).

The orthodontist treating patients with CPO should always be aware of their vertical growth pattern and the greater tendency towards relapse because of the palatal scar tissue.

Conclusion

Orthodontic treatment for children with clefts should:

- achieve an optimal occlusion and dentofacial aesthetics within the constraints imposed by the underlying skeletal pattern
- keep the duration of treatment to a minimum
- accomplish as much as possible during periods of active treatment
- be sympathetic to individual needs and circumstances
- make provision for assistance in maintaining good oral hygiene.

References and Bibliography

Action for Sick Children (1996) *Health Services for Children and Young People; A Guide for Commissioners and Providers: Principles for Commissioning and Providing Service*. Action for Sick Children, London: 5

Advanced Life Support Group (1997) *Advanced Paediatric Life Support: The Practical Approach*. BMJ Books, London: 9; 66

Avedian LV, Ruberg RL (1980). Impaired weight gain in cleft lip and palate infants. *Cleft Lip Palate J* **17**(1): 24–26

Andreasen JO (1992) *Atlas of Replantation and Transplantation of Teeth*. Mediglobe, Fribourg:

Ardveson JC (1993) *Pediatric Feeding and Swallowing*. Whurr Publishers, London

Armstrong AJ, Finch RG, Bailey FB (1993) Serious group A Streptococcal infections complicating cryotherapy to lip haemangiomas. *Clin Exp Dermatol* **18**: 537

Bagatin M (1985) Submucous cleft palate. *J Oral Maxillo-facial Surg* **13**(1): 37–38

Bannister RP (2001) Early feeding management. In: Watson ACH, Sell D, Grunwell P, eds. *Management of Cleft Lip and Palate*. Whurr Publishing, London: 137–47

Bath AP, Bull PD (1997) The Management of upper airway obstruction in Pierre Robin sequence. *J Laryngol Otology* **111**: 1155; 1157

Bergland O, Semb G, Byholm FE (1986) Elimination of the residual alveolar cleft by secondary bone grafting and subsequent orthodontic treatment. *Cleft Palate J* **23**: 175–205

Bergland O, Sidhu SS (1974) Occlusal changes from the deciduous to the early mixed dentition in unilateral complete clefts. *Cleft Palate J* **11**: 317–26

Berkowitz S (1994) *The Cleft Palate Story*. Quintessence Publishing, Chicago: 79

Black FB, Jarman L, Simpson JB (1998) *The Science of Breast Feeding*. Jones and Bartlett Publishers, Massachusetts: 86

Bøhn A (1963) Dental anomalies in harelip and cleft palate. *Acta Odontal Scand* **21**: 1–109

Bosworth C (1997) *Burns Trauma Nursing Procedures*. Whurr Publishing, London: 229

Boyne PJ, Sands NR (1976) Combined orthodontic-surgical management of residual palato-alveolar cleft defect. *Am J Orthod* **70**: 20–37

Brine EA, Rickard KA, Brady MS *et al* (1994) The effectiveness of two feeding methods in improving the energy and growth of infants with cleft lip and palate. A randomised study. *J Am Dietet Ass* **94**(7): 732–38

Brown J (1972) Instrumental control of sucking response in newborns. *J Exp Psychol* 14: 66–88

Bu Lock F, Woolridge MW, Baum JD (1990) Development of co-ordination of breathing, sucking and swallowing. *Child Neurol* **32**: 669–78

Burdi AR (1969) Sexual differences in closure of the human palatal shelves. *Cleft Palate J* **6**: 1

Changing Faces Publications, 1–2 Junction Mews, London, W2 1PN; *Psychoanalytic Child* **17**: 245–64

Chapple JR, Nunn JH (2001) The oral health of children with clefts of the lip, palate or both. *Cleft Palate Craniofac J* **38**: 525–28

Choi BH, Kleinhheinz J, Joos U, Komposch G (1991) Sucking efficiency of early orthopaedic plate and teats in infants with a cleft lip and palate. *Int J Oral Maxillofac Surg* **20**: 167–69

CLAPA in Association with Fetal Medicine Unit, St. Georges Hospital, London (2001) *Cleft Lip and Palate Guide for Sonographers*. Cleft Lip and Palate Association, London

Cleft Lip and Palate Association. Feeding Bottles and Teats Catalogue, 3rd Floor, 235-237 Finchley Rd, London NW7 6LD

Clifford E, Crocker G (1971) Maternal response: The birth of a normal child as compared to the birth of a child with a cleft. *Cleft Palate J* **8**: 298–306

Clinical Standards Advisory Group (CSAG) (1998) *Cleft Lip and/or Palate*. Report of a CSAG Committee. The Stationary Office, London

References

Coma Report (1994) *Weaning and the Weaning Diet.* Report on Health and Social Subjects 45. HMSO, London

Cowan DC, Kerr AIG (1986) Secretory otitis media. In: Birrell JF, ed. *Paediatric Otolaryngology.* Wright Publishers, Bristol: 145–48

Croen LA, Wasserman CR, Tolarová MM (1998) Racial and ethnic variations in the prevalence of orofacial clefts in California. *Am J Medic Gen* **79**: 42–47

Cuthbert AM (1994) Cleft Lip and Palate Survey; an Examination of 16 Hospitals Protocols for Cleft Lip and Palate Surgery. Unpublished, Royal Victoria Hospital, Newcastle. Sept to Dec

Dahl E (1970) Craniofacial morphology in congenital clefts of the lip and palate. An x-ray cephalometric study of young males. Dissertation. *Acta Odontol Scand* **28**(suppl): 57

Department of Health (2000) *Modernising Dietary Implementing the NHS Plan.* HMSO, London

Department of Health (1998) *Health Service Circular 1998/238, Cleft Lip and Palate Services—Commissioning Specialised Services.* DoH, London

Department of Health (1996) *The Patients Charter: Services for Children and Young People, and My Rights.* DoH, London

Department of Health (1991) *Welfare of Children and Young People in Hospital* (Guidance Document). HMSO, London: 16

Derijcke A, Eerens A, Carels C (1996) The incidence of oral clefts: A review. *Br J Oral Maxillofacial Surg* **34**: 488–94

Drotar D (1975) Adaption of parents to the birth of an infant with congenital abnormalities. *Pediatrics* **56**(5): 710–17

Dunstan SP, Korezak PK (1996) Use of epidural catheter for postoperative pain relief for bone harvesting from iliac crest. *Br J Oral Maxillofac Surg* **34**: 436–37

Enderby P (1986) Speech and language handicap: Towards knowing the size of the problem. *Br J Disord Communic* **21**:151–65

Enemark H, Bolund S, Jørgensen I (1990) Evaluation of unilateral cleft lip and palate treatment: Long-term results. *Cleft Palate J* **27**: 354–61

Enemark H, Sindet-Pedersen S, Bundgaard M (1987) Long-term results after secondary bone grafting of alveolar clefts. *J Oral Maxillofac Surg* **45**: 913–18

Erwin EC, MacWilliams BJ (1973) Parents working with parents: The cleft palate program. *Cleft Palate J* **10**: 360–66

Farrell M, Holder S (1992) Familial recurrence pattern analysis of cleft lip with or without cleft palate. *Am J Hum Genet* **50**: 270–77

Golding-Kushner (2001) *Therapy Techniques for Cleft Palate Speech and Related Disorders*. Singular Publishers, London

Gollup R (1997) Burns aftercare and scar management. In: Bosworth C, ed. *Burns Trauma*. Balliere Tindall, London: 165

Gorlin RJ, Cohen MM, Hennekam RCM (2001) Syndromes of the head and neck. In: *Orofacial Clefting Syndromes: General Aspects*. Oxford University Press, Oxford: Ch 20

Grunwell P, Sell D (2001) Speech and cleft palate/velopharyngeal anomalies. In: Watson A, Sell D, Grunwell P, eds. *Management of Cleft Lip and Palate*. Whurr Publishing, London: 68–87

Harding A, Grunwell P (1996) Characteristics of cleft palate speech. *Eur J Disord Communic* **31**(4): 331–57

Harding A, Harland K, Razzell R (1997) *Cleft Audit Protocol for Speech (CAPS)*. Available from: SLT Dept, St Andrews Centre for Plastic Surgery, Broomfield Hospital, Court Rd, Broomfield, Chelmsford, Essex, UK

Harper PS (2003) *Practical Genetic Counselling*, 5th edn. Butterworth Heineman, Oxford

Herzog-Isler C (1994) Video Showing Breast Fed Infants with Cleft Lip and Palate, Pilatus Strasse 4 Ch-6033 Buchrain, Switzerland

Herzog-Isler C, Honigmann K (1996) *Give Us a Little Time*. Medela AG, Switzerland

Isolauri E, Arvola T, Sütas Y, Moilanen E, Salminen S (2000) Probiotics in the management of eczema. *Clin Exper Allergy* **30**(11): 1604–10

Itikala PR, Watkins ML, Mulinare J, Moore CA, Lui Y (2001) Maternal multivitamin use and orofacial clefts in offspring. *Teratology* **63**(2): 79–86

Jiginni V, Kangesu T, Sommerlad BC (1993) Do babies require arm splints after cleft palate repair? *Br J Plastic Surg* **46**: 681–85

References

Johnston MC, Sulik KK (1979) Some abnormal patterns of development in the craniofacial region. *Birth Defects* **15**(8): 23–42

Jones E, Dimmock P, Spencer SA (2001) Randomised controlled trial to compare methods of milk expression following pre-term delivery. *Arch Dis Child* **85F**: 91–95

Jones KL (1997) *Smith's Recognizable Patterns of Human Malformation*. WB Saunders Company, Philadelphia

Jones WB (1988) Weight gain and feeding in the neo-natal with a cleft: A 3 centre study. *Cleft Palate J* **25**(4): 379–84

Kennedy I (2001) *The Bristol Royal Infirmary Inquiry*. Department of Health, London

Kent R (2002) Nasogastric Feeding Post Palate Repair—An Option. Paper presented at Nurses Special Interest Group, *Craniofacial Society Annual Conference*, East Grinstead

Kowash M (2000) Effectiveness on oral health. Education programme for mothers with young children. *Br Dental J* **188**: 201–205

Kono D, Young L, Holtman B (1981) The association of submucous cleft palate and clefting of the primary palate. *Cleft Palate J* 18(3): 207–209

Kubler Ross E (1970) Grief and loss. *Psychoanal Study Child* 16: 6–24

Lax R (1972) Some aspects of the interaction between mother and the impaired child. *Int JPsychoanalysis* **55**: 339–43

Lees M (2001) Genetics of cleft lip and palate. In: Watson ACH, Sell D, Grunwell P, eds. *Management of Cleft Lip and Palate*. Whurr Publishers, London: 87–104

Lello GE (2001) Orthognathic surgery. In: Watson ACH, Sell DA, Grunwell P, eds. *Management of Cleft Lip and Palate*. Whurr Publishers, London: Ch 21; 338–51

Lennox P (2001) Hearing and ENT management. In: Watson ACH, Sell D, Grunwell P, eds. *Management of Cleft Lip and Palate*. Whurr Publishers, London: 213

Majamaa H, Isolauri E (1997) Probiotics: a novel approach in the management of food allergy. *J Allergy Clin Immun* **99**(2): 179–85

Manolson A (1992) *It Takes Two to Talk: A Hanen Early Language Parent Guide Book*. Winslow Press, Oxford

Mars M (2001) Alveolar bone grafting. In: Watson ACH, Sell D, Grunwell P, eds. *Management of Cleft Lip and Palate*. Whurr Publishers, London: Ch 20; 326–37

Martin V (2002) Evaluation of Different Feeding Methods for Children with a Cleft Lip and/or Palate. Thesis, Nottingham University

Martin V (2001) Pre and post operative nursing care. In: Watson ACH, Sell D, Grunwell P, eds. *Management of Cleft Lip and Palate*. Whurr Publishers, London: 184–190

Martin V (1999) Cleft lip and palate: reflections on a Nepaly experience. *Paediatr Nurs* **11**(6): 6–8

Martin V, Abbett M (2003) *Feeding your Baby with a Cleft Lip and/or Palate—Your Options*. Central Medical Supplies Publication, Leek, Staffordshire

Martin V, Henley M, Rose DH (unpublished). In Utero Diagnosis for Cleft Lip and Palate in Mid-Trent, UK—Developing Support for the Family, Nottingham Cleft Team, Nottingham

Millard DR, jnr (1980) *Cleft Craft*, Vol III. Little, Brown and Company, Boston

Miller M (1994) The ideal healing environment. *Nurs Times* 90: 62–68

Morley M (1970) *Cleft Palate Speech*. Churchill Livingstone, Edinburgh, London and New York

Newman J (2000) *Breast Compression*. Handout 15. Website: www.bflrc.com/newman/articles.htm

Nottingham City Hospital (1994) *Parent Information Booklet: Hello, My Name is Jade*. Nottingham City Hospital NHS Trust: p3.10

Paradise JL, Elster BA, Tan L (1994) Evidence of infants with cleft palate that breast milk protects against otitis media. *Paediatrics* **94**(6): 853–54

Patten Bradley M (1976) *Patten's Human Embryology*. McGraw-Hill Book Company, New York and London

Phillips S, Dayborn AK, Hatch DJ (1994). Pre-operative fasting for paediatric anaesthesia. *Br J Anaesth* **73**: 529–36

Powell L (1998) Caries prediction: A review of the literature. *Commun Dent Oral Epidemiol* **26**: 361–71

References

Proffit WR (1993) *Contemporary Orthodontics*. Mosby–Year Book, St Louis

Ranta R (1986) A review of tooth formation in children with cleft lip/palate. *Am J Orthod* **90**: 11–18

Rifkin CJ, Keith O, Crawford PJM, Mathorn IS (2000) Dental care of the patient with a cleft lip and palate, part I. *Br Dental J* **188**(2): 78–83; Dental care part 2. *Br Dental J* **188**(3): 131–34

Roberts E, Kallen B, Harris J (1996) The epidemiology of orofacial clefts. 1. Some general epidemiological characteristics. *J Craniofacial Gen Develop Biol* **16**(4): 234–41

Robertson J (1962) Mothering as an Influence on Early Development. *Psychoanal Study Child* **17**: 245–64

Robson AK, Blanchard JD, Jones K, Albery EH, Smith IM, Maw AR (1992) A conservative approach to the management of otitis media with effusion in cleft palate children. *J Laryngol Otology* **106**: 788–92

Roch WP (1994) Young children and fluoride toothpaste. *Br Dental J* **177**: 17–20

Rollnick BR, Pruzansky S (1981) Genetic services at a centre for craniofacial anomalies. *Cleft Palate J* **18**: 304–13

Ross RB, Johnston MC (1972) *Cleft Lip and Palate*. Williams and Wilkins, Baltimore

Royal College of Obstetricians and Gynaecologists (2000) *Routine Ultrasound Screening in Pregnancy. Protocol, Standards and Training*. RCOG Press, London

Royal College of Paediatrics and Child Health (1997) *Prevention and Control of Pain in Children: a Manual for Health Care Professionals*. BMJ Books, London: 55;124

Russell VJ, Harding A (2001) Speech development and early intervention. In: Watson A, Sell D, Grunwell P, eds. *Management of Cleft Lip and Palate*. Whurr Publishers, London: 191–210

Saavedra JM, Bauman NA, Oung I, Perman JA, Yolken RH (1994) Feeding of Bifidobacterium bifidum and streptococcus thermophilus to infants in hospital for prevention of diarrhoea and shedding of rotavirus. *Lancet* **344**(October 15): 1046–49

Schechter GL (1990) Physiology of the mouth, pharynx and oesophagus. In: Bluestone CD, ed. *Paediatric Otolaryngology*. WB Saunders, Philadelphia: 816

Seligman MEP (1975) *Helplessness*. Freeman, San Francisco

Sell D, Harding A, Grunwell P (1999) P. GOS.SP.ASS. '98: An assessment for speech disorders associated with cleft palate and/or velopharyngeal dysfunction (revised). *Int J Lang Communic Disord* **34**(1): 17–33

Semb G, Shaw WC (2001) Orthodontics. In: Watson ACH, Sell DA, Grunwell P, eds. *Management of Cleft Lip and Palate*. Whurr Publishers, London: Ch 19; 299–325

Semb G, Shaw WC (1996) Facial growth in orofacial clefting disorders. In: Turvey TA, Vig KWL, Fonseca RJ, eds. *Facial Clefts and Craniosynostosis. Principles and Management*. WB Saunders, Philadelphia: Ch 2; 28–56

Serra AM, Bailey CM, Jackson P (1986) *Ear Nose and Throat Nursing*. Blackwell Scientific Publications, Oxford: 230

Seth AK, McWilliams BJ (1988) Weight gain in children with cleft palate from birth to two years. *Cleft Palate J* **25**: 146–50

Shaw WC (1993) *Orthodontics and Occlusal Management*. Butterworth-Heinemann, Oxford

Shaw WC, Asher-McDade C, Brattström DDS *et al* (1992) A six-centre international study of treatment outcomes in patients with clefts of the lip and palate. *Cleft Palate Craniofac J* **29**(5): 393–418

Shaw WC, Bannister RP, Roberts CT (1999) Assisted feeding is more reliable for infants with clefts. *Craniofac J* **36**(3): 262–68

Shprintzen R (1988) Pierre Robin, micrognathia and airway obstruction the dependency of treatment of accurate diagnosis. *Int Anaesth Clin* **26**: 64–67

Shprintzen RJ, Schwatz RH, Daniller A, Hoch L (1985) Morphologic significance of bifid uvula. *Paediatrics* **75**: 553–61

Shprintzen RJ, Siegel-Sladewitz VL, Amato J, Goldberg RB (1985) Anomalies associated with cleft lip, cleft palate or both. *Am J Medic Genet* **20**: 585–96

Solnit A, Stark MH (1962), Mourning and the birth of a defective child. *Psychoanal Study Child* **16**: 523–37

References

Stebbens VA, Poets CF, Alexander JR, Arrowsmith WA, Southall DP (1991) Oxygen saturations and breathing patterns in infancy: 1. Full term infants in the second month of life. *Arch Dis Child* **66**: 569–73

Tolarova M, Harris J (1995) Reduced recurrence of orofacial clefts after periconceptional supplementation with high-dose folic acid and multivitamins. *Teratol* **51**(2): 71–78

Turner MM, Milward TM (1988) A study to assess the effectiveness of a professional and lay support service for parents of new born cleft babies. *Br J Plastic Surg* **41**: 614–18

Twycross A, Moriarty A, Betts T (1998) *Paediatric Pain Management—A Multi-Disciplinary Approach*. Radcliffe Medical Press, Oxford: 128–29

UNICEF UK. Baby Friendly Initiative Leaflet, Breast Feeding Your Baby. UNICEF Enterprises Ltd

United Kingdom Association of Sonographers (2001) Guidelines for Professional Working Standards—Ultrasound Practice

Ward S (2000) Baby Talk. Random House, London and New York

Watson ACH, Sell D, Grunwell P, eds (2001) *Management of Cleft Lip and Palate*. Whurr Publishing, London

Whether F, Woolridge MW, Baum JD (1986) An ultrasonographic study of the organisation of sucking and swallowing by newborn infants. *Develop Med Child Neurol* **28**: 19–24

Winnicott DW (1987) *Home is Where We Start*. Penguin Books, Harmondsworth

Woolridge MW (1986) Anatomy of infant sucking. *Midwif* **2**(4): 164–71

Woolridge MW, Fisher C (1988), Overfeeding and symptoms of lactose malabsorption. *Lancet* **2**: 382–83

Yaster M, Maxwell LG (1993) Opiate agonists and antagonists. In: Schecter NL, Berde CB, Yaster M, eds. *Pain in Infants, Children and Adolescents*. Williams and Wilkins, Baltimore: 145–71

Index

Index

Index